A Guide For Bereaved Parents
Who Are Making Decisions
About Their Future

155,937
SCH

193 2480

by

Pat Schwiebert, RN
Co-Founder and Professional Liaison,
Compassionate Friends, Portland (Oregon) Chapter

Director, Perinatal Loss
Oregon Health Sciences University Foundation

Paul Kirk, MD
Professor and Chairman,
Department of Obstetrics and Gynecology
Oregon Health Sciences University

1

Dedication

This book is written in memory of those
infants who have lived very short lives
but who have made a big impact on the quality
of the lives of others.

Blake Delaney, son of Melissa and Joe Delaney
Mariah McNassar Stewart, daughter of Kathy McNassar and Randy Stewart
Benjamin Marx, son of Gary and Maggie Marx
Micalee Swanton, daughter of Peggy and Larry Swanton
Jana and Joel Powers, children of Joanna and Jim Powers
Cedar Kerr-Valentic, daughter of Judy and Frank Kerr-Valentic
Holly Stanbro, daughter of Mike and Barbara Stanbro
Joseph and Thomas Packard, sons of Laurie and Rick Packard
Katie Sandberg, daughter of Bea and Chris Sandberg
Nicolas Shearer, son of Bob and Debbie Shearer
Keith Castlio, son of Cheryl and Mike Castlio
Shawn Arsenault, son of Linda and Russ Arsenault
Emily Johnson, daughter of Evelyn Taylor and Jeff Johnson
Alexander and Celeste Still, children of Susan and Gene Still
Anna and Ben Olson, children of Molly and Rob Olson

Table of Contents

Foreword

This book has not been an easy one to write. There were times when we questioned putting it into print because parts of it sounded so negative. We too found ourselves caught in the "if-we-don't-talk-about-it-then-it-doesn't-exist" trap.

We would rather have been able to write something that could assure you that your life will be easier after the tragedy you have endured, but the painful truth is that your life won't be easy — at least not for a while. Just like taking prepared childbirth classes didn't prevent you from feeling the pain of birth, neither will this book make it unnecessary for you to experience grief, fear or ambivalence during a subsequent pregnancy. Facing that truth is an important part of the healing process, and that, in part, is what we offer to you in this book.

We hope that as you read this book you will respond in either of two ways. On the one hand you may develop a case of the "uh huhs," because you too have thought similar thoughts. Or perhaps you will feel relieved as you discover that your subsequent pregnancy isn't as worrisome as most, after all.

Chapter 1
After A Loss

Dear Katie,

I wanted so much to keep you
that I thought getting pregnant
would help. Instead this pregnancy has left
me torn. So many things are becoming
clear lately. Slowly, very slowly,
your death is becoming a reality.
I loved you and still do . . . so much
I just couldn't face your not
being with me. But you are gone,
and I will survive, as will your
memory.

I am forced now, more than before, to
say goodbye. Your sister or brother
is now joining our lives and I must
make room for this new individual.

Your book is complete, my love.
Life, Birth, Death. For you it was
very quick . . . too quick.
It is goodbye for now. Only for now
I say, "Goodbye, my child."

> *With all my love,*
>
> *Your mother*
> *Bea Sandberg*

You just had a wonderful visit with a friend who you know you are not going to see again for a long time. Just as you are about to say your goodbyes some other good friend that you've been anxious to see arrives. Your loyalties are divided. Your goodbyes with your friend are shortened. You find it difficult to immediately transfer your thoughts and interest to your newly arrived guest; you find yourself still preoccupied with the first visitor.

If we are to admit that our past experiences have a profound effect on how we now live and act, then we must assume that a parent who has experienced the death of a child will find her future childbearing and childrearing experiences different from those of her "untouched" sisters. For this reason *Still To Be Born* needed to be written.

As families plod along the lonely road of grief after the death of their babies, it becomes obvious that the process is incomplete until the parents come to grips with two questions: "Shall we have another baby?" and, if yes, "When?"

Most of us caring, but naive, friends and professionals have had no idea how difficult it is for bereaved parents to make such decisions. The lack of understanding that has led us in the past to encourage bereaved parents to deny the death of their newborn child, continues to be reflected in our attempts to be helpful in this new situation.

We have offered well-meaning, but inappropriate, advice: "Try again . . . you just had bad luck."

We, the authors of this book, might still be making these mistakes ourselves were it not for the lessons which bereaved parents have taught us. It is their teaching which has inspired this book.

Bereaved parents come to Compassionate Friends meetings to share their grief with others. They talked about their dead babies, their own anguish, their anger that such a tragedy could have been dealt to them, their fears that it could happen again, and their hope that they would be able to regain some sort of control in their lives. Each time a bereaved family revealed that they were pregnant again there were mixed reactions from others in the group. Most of the parents were genuinely pleased for the newly pregnant couples. But at the same time the others were also being reminded that they did not have such good news to share; to them, that pregnant woman sitting next to them had become an outsider.

The pregnant woman, in turn, began to feel like an intruder in a group that once brought her great comfort. She felt a sense of guilt as she tried to make conversation with her not-so-lucky sisters. Already isolated from those who had never experienced the death of a child, she now also felt isolated from those who had known a similar grief experience, but who had not yet faced the challenge of a subsequent pregnancy. She needed persons whom she could trust to understand and accept her ambivalent feelings in this new situation.

We created a subsequent pregnancy support group four years ago to meet the needs of those who had "outgrown" Compassionate Friends, but still needed a support network in their new situation. This book contains teachings from the members of that group who dared to admit what it felt like inside the body of a mother waiting for someone to mother.

The intent of this book is to help validate feelings bereaved parents may experience during a subsequent pregnancy, to give some suggestions on how they may cope in their new situation, and to offer these same parents some hope for the future.

As you read this book, don't assume that all the feelings expressed are those that every parent will experience. Notice how different some reactions will be from others, even though the experiences which prompted them appear to be quite similar. There are no "right" ways.

When your infant dies your future is put on hold until you can come to terms with your past.

Are You Still Grieving For Your Dead Child?

When bereaved persons are asked how long they think it will take for them to get over their grief they will usually answer, "Forever." These are people who have endured the loss of something special to them. They are speaking from experience.

Those who have never had to suffer the intense pains of

loss tend to underestimate the time required for "grief work" to be completed. That is because they are projecting an assumption based upon their own limited experience, for indeed it does not take long for them to "get over" someone else's loss.

The same is true, but to a lesser extent, where friends and relations — other than a spouse or child — are involved. Most people find that it takes no more than from forty-eight hours to two weeks to get their lives back to a normal routine after suffering the death of a close friend or relative not in the immediate nuclear family.

For bereaved parents, however, the readjustment of one's life following a loss of a child takes approximately eighteen to twenty-four months. This does not mean that after twenty-four months the death is forgotten; it simply means that this much time is needed to come to terms with the loss.

Two years seems like an incredibly long time to have to suffer the pains of grief. And so it is, as any bereaved parent will testify. Fortunately, the intensity of the grief does subside somewhat after the first month, but the continuing process of putting one's life back together after such a loss will still be filled with many bewildering moments.

If you are a newly bereaved parent, you may find after a few months that you are really tired of being depressed, and weary of not having the energy or enthusiasm to enjoy life. You may be afraid you will always feel this bad and — at the same time — be afraid that you will not feel bad enough and so appear to be disloyal to your dead child. It's not easy to be in the body of the bereaved.

Grief over the death of your own infant is the loneliest of all griefs. This is especially true if your child died at birth or shortly after because no one else besides you has any memories about the child to cling to or to share. No one else had the same hopes and aspirations for this child's future nor did they make changes in their lives to accommodate this new person.

Don't be surprised if you find yourself feeling angry at the lack of sensitivity of others to your need for continued acknowledgement of your dead baby. You may think it's only fair that they suffer as much as you are suffering over your loss. But they simply can't do it. And it's unrealistic as well as unfair to think they will. Most likely if you were to find that others were grieving as much as you, or showing more outward grief over your child than you, you would be just as upset and angry. Remember, it was your unique relationship with your child that made your future so hopeful, and that now makes your grief so intense. No one else can feel your grief as keenly as you do.

There will be a few people in your life who will be able to accommodate your needs and be there for you. You'll know who they are. They are the ones who won't try to change the subject when you need to talk about your baby. Take advantage of their caring, and be grateful for them.

In the case of a miscarriage most people, unless they know that you were pregnant, will be totally unaware of your loss. It will be impossible for them to support you unless you share what's happened in your life, and express to others your feelings of loss.

When an older child dies, family and friends will have a greater feeling of loss, because the child did make an impact on them also. Special times will be remembered, and "videotapes" will play in their heads reminding them of "precious moments." Even if an older dead child is not mentioned (often because other family members and friends are uncomfortable, or don't want to upset the bereaved parents) the parents at least know that this child was a part of others' lives, and that the child is remembered by them.

The first year following an infant's death is filled with important anniversaries of "first times" and "missed times" — the first Christmas you had looked forward to celebrating with your baby, the first spring day, your first trip to the beach. Everything you do will remind you that you had earlier planned to do it with your baby. As the anniversary of your pregnancy comes around you will be aware that it was at this or that specific time one year ago that the first sign of trouble appeared, or that the baby was "due", or was born, or died.

Indeed if you find yourself wondering why you are having a particularly difficult time, it may be because you are subconsciously aware of some anniversary associated with your dead baby's life. The unconscious mind will play funny games with your breaking heart reminding you not to forget. It is helpful to keep track of those special dates so you can use them well to remember your time with and feelings about your baby.

The brain gives up a lot less easily than the body
Norman Maclean

"If it weren't for the unique and innate relationship between parent and child that says 'I love you no matter what,' some babies would never come home from the hospital."

Why Grieve For Someone You Didn't Know?

Does the following sound familiar? Has something like this happened to you?

The grace period lasted about a month. During this time our friends accepted or at least tolerated our grief.

After a month they began to send us subtle messages: "It's time to move on with life," or "you should be over your sadness by now." Whenever we would mention our dead baby by name, or speak of the child in normal conversation, our well-meaning friends would scramble for an excuse to change the subject.

These friends seemed to deny our need to grieve over the loss of this child by making statements like these: "You're young. You can always have another baby," or "It won't happen again."

We were made to feel uncomfortable because we continued to have this strong feeling of love for a person who, in the eyes of our friends, no longer existed. We were sometimes embarrassed by the intensity of our emotions when we remembered this child who was but a phantom to others. We found it harder to justify our feelings about this child than if, at the time of his death, he had been old enough to be known and remembered by others.

As a society we seem to be sending a double message to you who are bereaved parents. Before the death, we talked about how important this child was — a part of our hope for the future of the race, a gift to be cared for and loved. Now we expect you to quickly dismiss and forget this same child as no longer important. But something prevents you from abandoning the memory of this little one.

We easily forget that this child was an integral part of your personal future and therefore not a person to be casually discarded. The fact that others have also lost children has no bearing on your pain. Your pain is your own and can't be compared with the pain of anyone else.

During the past few years much attention has been given to the attachment process that takes place between parent and child at birth, and to the importance of those first few moments together for cementing that relationship. Though bonding has been emphasized as a dynamic in the birth process we also know that you were busy during the prenatal period establishing an important parent-child relationship.

If there had been no bonding taking place between you and your child prenatally then there would be no grief for you to endure post-partum. The death of your child could then be experienced as a minor disappointment and a very temporary disruption in your lives. But because of the bonding process, your unborn child was a part of your lives in a very real way, even though you never "met" in the usual sense. Therefore, the loss of your child is profound, the grief deep and the adjustment process difficult. Grief over the loss of your baby is a beautiful statement to your child that "I loved you all of your life."

You will read examples of parents who actually did try to protect themselves from possible future pain in a subsequent pregnancy by keeping the new unborn child at a safe emotional distance, unconsciously trying not to bond so that they would not have to risk grief again. Though this may seem like a reasonable approach, the parent-child relationship in the subsequent pregnancy is handicapped by the resistance to the normal, natural bonding process. On a more positive note, as surely as love goes, no matter how hard you may try to hold your love back, you can't help falling in love with your little one.

As for me
I would rather be able to love
things I cannot have,
Than to have things
I'm not able to love.
Merrit Malloy

Time Alone Does Not Heal

Use your time well. Don't just go home from the hospital after your baby has died and pretend that nothing has happened. You know something has happened. Acknowledge it. Let yourself feel the pain of caring. That's the price a person must be willing to pay for love.

Here are some things you can do to help yourself resolve some of the feelings you are likely to have after your baby has died.

1. Talk to your doctor about what actually happened. If there was an autopsy done have the findings explained to you. Your labor and delivery nurse may be able to help you remember things you can't remember.

2. Seek genetic counseling if that is appropriate in your situation. Find out about the statistical probabilities of this happening to you again.

3. Make a scrap book or special box where you can keep things that will help you remember your baby's short life with you. (Pictures, mementos from the birth, prenatal visits, current events, thoughts you had about this child.)

4. Talk with others about how you are feeling. If there is a Compassionate Friends, SHARE or AMEND group in your area, get in touch with these people. (Refer to page 117 for addresses.) All of these people know what it's like to have a baby die. They can help you understand and accept your feelings. It has been said that 50% of all stress is relieved by talking things over with someone else.

5. Talk with your partner. Let each other know what you are feeling. Don't assume that you are both on the same grief schedule.

6. Start a diary. Write about what you are thinking now. This will be helpful to you. Months from now as you look back you'll see how far you have come.

7. Exercise. Physical activity is a very important means to reduce stress. Go on long walks, or sign up for an exercise or dance class. Such activity will improve not only your physical well being, but your mental health as well.

8. Be kind to yourself. Look for ways to reduce stress in your life. For example, if you get upset because the dishes don't get done after dinner, but you lack the energy to tackle the job yourself, offer to pay a teenager in your neighborhood to come in nightly to help out.

9. Don't take medications that may be detrimental to a pregnancy if you are planning to conceive soon.
10. Practice birth control until you are sure you want to get pregnant again.

Have you come to the Red Sea place in your life
Where, in spite of all you can do,
There is no way out, there is no way back,
There is no other way but through?

Annie Johnson Flint

SOME TRAVELING MUSIC

How can you say something new
  about being alone?
Tell someone you're a loner
and right away they think you're lonely.

It's not the same thing, you know.

It's not wanting to put all your marbles
  in one pocket.
It's caring enough not to care too much.

Mostly it's letting yourself come first for a while.

— *Rod McKuen*

Melissa's Story

"Walking on a thin sheet of ice" — that's the best way to describe those nine long months of my pregnancy with Devin. I was afraid to grieve for Blake for fear of upsetting myself and then possibly hurting this pregnancy. I now wonder if I was using this new pregnancy as an excuse to put off my mourning Blake's death. I promised myself that I would deal with his death at a later date. But right now, I needed to make me a baby.

I was obsessed with getting pregnant. It was on my mind all the time. Every time I started my period I cried. It was just another example of what a failure I was. I wasn't grieving for my son. I was grieving because I wasn't pregnant. I charted my temperature carefully while I waited anxiously for the sign that I was ovulating. There was no joy in our lovemaking. Intercourse was merely a means to an end.

Two long months had come and gone since Blake's birth and death day. I was due for my postpartum check up. Though we had used an in home pregnancy test kit and the test turned out negative I was sure that I was pregnant. I just had to be! The doctor arranged for a blood test to see if my intuition was correct.

Since it was Friday I would have to wait until Monday before hearing the test results. But when the nurse called on Monday to report the good news she encountered only dead silence from my end of the phone. She wasn't any more surprised than I was at my ambiguous reaction. I too had expected that I would be overcome with joy. Instead I hung up the phone and cried for at least a lifetime. The fear I felt was overwhelming. I was afraid of being hurt again and afraid of being a traitor to Blake's memory.

How grateful I was that my doctor sensed my anxieties about this pregnancy and suggested that we schedule more frequent visits. I don't think I would have had the nerve to ask for them myself. I was afraid others would think I was asking for favors and overreacting.

As luck would have it fetal heart tones couldn't be heard at the expected time and we were sent to have an ultrasound done. Back I went to the same office, the same room where I had gone during pregnancies past. My thoughts were centered on Blake. Why hadn't this radiologist detected Blake's heart problem and warned me so I could have prepared myself for his death? I had convinced myself that I was not going to cry and make a scene. Somehow I managed to blurt out Blake's story and my sense of foreboding about this new baby, without being consumed in tears.

This doctor was like a gift from heaven. He spent a lot of time talking with me about Blake. He explained that Blake's heart problem couldn't have been detected prior to his birth. He also assured me that as far as he could tell this new baby was developing well. Fetal heart tones could be both seen and heard. What a relief. I wanted so much to believe the doctor's assurances that all was well.

Months five and six were pretty good. Cautiously optimistic, we purchased a new crib and high chair. The crib was stored in the garage, but the high chair became a trophy in our kitchen just waiting to be awarded. This was to be our reminder that we had to think positively about this pregnancy.

I rationalized that if this baby died, I would accept the death bravely, and I would just keep having babies until I had one that lived. After all, I couldn't possibly hurt more than I already did.

During my seventh and eighth month I developed a deep concern about my own health. I had fears that I might die during delivery and never see this child. My fears were almost totally centered on myself and on the prospect of undergoing another cesarean section. My fears had no grounding whatsoever, although at times I felt almost paralyzed by those fears.

When I arrived home after each checkup others in our family would hover around me and ask all kinds of questions. The kids, it turned out, were also concerned about my health, and one day they even asked who would be their mother, if I died.

At the end of July I decided it was time to bring out the baby clothes and arrange the corner of the room that was designated for the new baby. I made sure to arrange it as differently as possible. As each little item was brought out I cried. They were meant for Blake. This pregnancy seemed so unnecessary.

I had already decided to make another more elaborate christening gown for this baby. But whenever I worked on it I would start to cry. I believed it had to be done on time — just in case.

Every day I would read the obituaries. I imagined that if another baby died immediately before I had mine then my

17

baby would live. And I checked to make sure that the space in the cemetery next to Blake's was vacant — just in case. I did a lot of bargaining with God.

My due date had been moved up two weeks. I began to wonder if I would keep my sanity, even with two less weeks to worry. The ice on which I was walking was getting very thin.

Then labor started prematurely. I was put on medication to stop the labor until tests could be done to see if the baby's lungs were mature. "Not yet," the doctor said. I remained in the labor room for three more days and continued to receive medication. Being in the labor room was like reliving a nightmare. Though the nurses were encouraging and understanding, I felt like I was just prolonging the inevitable. I was anxious to get it over with, but I was afraid of the outcome. I was grateful that my nurse made sure I didn't have to be in the same labor room where I had waited for Blake's arrival. Then I was sent back home for two more weeks of medication.

Another amniocentesis two weeks later revealed a baby ready to be born. Thank goodness. We were down to the finish, and I had managed to maintain my sanity. Sleep did not come easily the night before my cesarean section. Joe was beside me holding my hand as I was wheeled into surgery. We hardly spoke. Because I had to have a general anesthetic, I was unable to see the birth of my son. I was told Devin had a very slow start due to all the medication I had taken to delay labor.

Two days passed before I finally got to see Devin. Until then Joe would go into the NICU and take polaroid pictures and bring them back for me to see. When I first saw Devin, he took my breath away. He looked exactly like Blake, as I remembered him.

Another two days went by before we were informed by an intern that Devin had a heart murmur. It was like all the worst was now coming true. Joe almost fainted when he heard the words "heart murmur."

Our pediatrician was called to come to the hospital to explain things to us. A heart problem means death to us. That's been our experience. Now they're telling us Devin's heart is not so bad. Does this mean that we just have to wait a little longer before we have to go through that pain again?

Devin came home in my arms when he was seven days old. He was pink, alert, and eating well. Everything was normal. No problem. But his father reacted to his homecoming by breaking out in a rash all over his body. Joe blamed it on the soap I used to do the wash, though it was the same soap I had used for years. We both really knew it was because he was an emotional wreck.

Three and a half weeks after Devin was born we celebrated Blake's first birth and death day. I held Devin in my arms all day. I had believed that having the new baby would fill me with joy, but there I was, deep in sorrow for my dead son, Blake. I felt like a traitor. I missed Blake so much and wanted him with me.

I now agree that putting some space between a baby's death and another baby's birth makes sense. We've made it, that's true, and our new baby is a delight, but we would have been much kinder to ourselves if we had waited.

Melissa Delaney

Roadblocks to Grieving

Individuals grieve in their own time and in their own way. Sometimes there are factors that tend to delay or prevent people from grieving. Here is a list of roadblocks that interfere with the completion of the grief process:

1. A parent may assume that because she never saw the child, she hasn't really suffered a loss and therefore has no need to grieve. She pretends that nothing serious has happened and simply goes on with her life.
2. The parent may have so much anger, rejection or guilt about the loss that these feelings may prevent the parent from mourning her baby's death.
3. There may be a stigma attached to the loss. If the parent had an abortion, adopted the baby out, or terminated the pregnancy due to knowledge that there were going to be severe complications in the infant's health, the sense of shame may prevent the parent from disclosing her sorrow to others, with the result that she does not receive the needed acknowledgement and support from them.
4. The parent may not want to make others feel bad and therefore may hide or suppress expressions of grief.

5. If the parent suffered a previous loss, was overwhelmed by the intensity of grief and did not receive support, she may block out the experience of grief so as not to have to feel the pain again.
6. If a parent's whole life and future were dependent on this child, and if her personal identity was related primarily to her becoming a mother, she may have difficulty letting go because this would mean giving up her only source of self-esteem.
7. The parent may be afraid to let go for fear that the child will be forgotten.
8. The parent may be denied opportunities to talk about the dead child and to express grief openly.
9. Parents of multiple births, where one child lives and the other dies, may have difficulty in both attaching with the live baby and saying goodbye to the one(s) who died.
10. Parents who have a series of tragedies within a short period may have difficulty separating out the emotions for individual tragedies.

When you suppress or repress those things which you don't want to live with, you don't really solve the problem because you don't bury the problem dead . . . you bury it alive. It remains alive and active inside of you.

John Powell

OZ

I'm not looking for answers anymore,
But for something to remember.

Merrit Malloy

Letting Go

No doubt you have been told by well-meaning friends that you must let go of your grief and get on with life. They are anxious for you to find life beyond grief as soon as possible. What they want for you, however, is easier said than done. Our work with bereaved parents has shown us that though the process of letting go is important and necessary, it is also extremely difficult for most parents. It is not something that one should expect to achieve very early in the grief process.

What is "letting go," and how does one go about it? Letting go is simply reaching the point of being able to say, "I will release the grip that I have on the past. No longer will I cling to my desire to hold the child I cannot hold. Nor will I continue to deny the reality that I will never be able to diaper and to nurture the child and to offer the amenities that I always expected would be a part of my parenting of this child."

Letting go does not mean that I will forget my child. Letting go means only that I accept that my child really is dead and that no amount of wanting and yearning and thinking about my child will bring him back. Letting go is accepting life as it really is without pretending that I can make it otherwise. It is also deciding that I can indeed be a happy person with my new and different life. It's allowing yourself to reinvest your energy and interest into something or someone else.

Letting go means that I won't need to think of the child every single day in order to keep her memory alive. I will be satisfied with the past that I held with her. I will remember special times that I shared with this child, even if all I was able to share were times of kicking and hiccupping. For some mothers it is enough to remember fondly how they sat quietly in the rocking chair singing lullabies to an unborn child as they caressed their bulging bellies.

Some parents are afraid to let go for fear that this would indicate disloyalty to their child. They assume that if they no longer hurt then they are being unfaithful to their child's memory. If this is true in your case, you might find it helpful to focus on the quality of the memory rather than the need to hang on to the pain. Do you really think your child needs you to be sad for him? Remember, the only life your child will have in this world after his or her death is through the life that you live. You alone will carry this child's message. Whether it is to be a message of joy or gloom, hope or despair, is up to you.

As you read these words some of you may actually be angered to think that you are expected at some point to let go of your child. The idea of letting go may seem decidedly unparentlike. How could a caring parent, especially the parent of an infant, think of such a thing? When you are still picturing your child in a physical sense in this world, letting go seems synonymous with abandonment.

Actually letting go is very much consistent with parenting and it is anything but abandonment. Child psychologists understand that in every healthy relationship between parent and child there are points at which the parent "lets go" to allow the child the freedom he or she needs to develop into a unique individual. The process of letting go begins at birth and continues throughout the life of the child. The first time you allow someone else to care for your child in your absence, the first time they go to school, or the first time they go away for the weekend without you — these are all examples of "little let-goes" in a parent's life. Letting go of a child who has died should be seen as a continuation of this same process.

You yourself will decide when, and how much, you are willing to let go of your child and of your need to remain the nurturing parent of this child. You will decide when it is time to set your child free to be — apart from you — in your memory, acknowledging at the same time the new person you have become or will become because of the impact this child has made on your life. Before the death occurred you probably wanted nothing more than to be a good parent to the child. But since the plans have been changed, you are the one to decide if you will cling to the past, or accept the present reality and remain open to what lies ahead.

Our children will pass through our lives. Some may stay awhile, while others' journey through us will be brief. The time that we are given to be with our children is limited. They must leave. And we must let them go. But the time that we carry our children with us is forever, despite their leaving. Cherish the time we have.

For some parents, letting go will happen easily and naturally over a period of time. These parents will awaken one day to the awareness that the pain of their child's death has diminished. For some it will be religious faith that provides the strength and comfort to make the transition into a new life without the child. For others there will need to be a more conscious effort to let go.

It may be helpful for you to look at this period of transition as having three stages. The first stage is acknowledgement that with the death of your child there has come an ending to a part of your life. At first you will probably find yourself moving in and out of the denial that this is in fact true.

A typical denial scenario goes something like this: after you have gone home from the hospital, the phone rings. As you go to answer it you imagine that it is your doctor calling. You imagine that he is calling to tell you that there has been an unusual case of mistaken identity at the hospital. It was really another baby that died. Your baby is alive and healthy and waiting for you to come and take him to his new home.

Sometimes bereaved parents will imagine that they hear a baby crying even though the nursery is empty.

Such denial is natural, especially in the early stages of grief. But there is a need to move beyond denial to acceptance. Wrestling with your shattered reality, facing the agonizing truth that your baby is dead even though, by usual standards, he is much too young to die, and dealing with the sense that your own body has failed you — these are all ways of coming to terms with this ending in your life.

Don't just do something, sit there.

The second stage of this transition in your life is called the neutral zone. This is a period of nothingness, a time "between dreams" as William Bridges calls it in his book, *Transitions,* a time when the pressure is off for a while so that reseeding of your inner strengths can take place. During this time we urge you to find ways to be kind to yourself. Buy yourself a gift, or take an afternoon off and just play or read a book.

This is also an excellent time to reorganize your priorities, and to ask yourself, "What do I *really* want out of life?" Without thinking you may answer, "I want a baby, of course." But be honest with yourself. Do you want a baby now, or have you just programmed yourself to think that's what you want? Now that you have an opportunity to have more control on your future are you just blindly assuming this is your first choice, or are there some other possibilities that you might like to consider also?

Ask yourself another question: "If I died tomorrow, what would I regret not having accomplished?"

"The neutral zone is a great place to visit, but you wouldn't want to live there," says Bridges. There are people who do take up temporary residence in the neutral zone far longer than necessary. And why not? It's safe, pressure-free, demand-free. But it has no future. Try to think of the neutral zone as a crosswalk. Standing in the middle of the street for too long is a foolish thing to do. So is remaining in a long period of emptiness. The purpose of the neutral zone is to provide a connecting link between an ending and a new beginning.

Eventually you will be ready to undertake this new beginning. How will you know that the time has arrived? Most often it just happens. Things seem to fall into place, and if you are open and healed you'll seize the opportunity.

As you read this and apply it to your own situation you may already be pregnant. In other words you may have entered a new beginning phase without having experienced a prior ending or without having spent creative time in the neutral phase. When we allow new beginnings to come before endings it is usually because we are afraid of being left with nothing. Therefore we try to protect ourselves by having a substitute waiting in the wings. Or perhaps the reason is that we haven't been aware of the value of this three step process.

One problem with reversing the process is that we may find ourselves building our future on our unhealed past rather than on a past that has been resolved. For example, if a woman hates doctors because her baby died and she hasn't worked that feeling through, it will be very difficult for her to trust a doctor during her next pregnancy. If she thinks she is marked by fate and that her tragedy will be repeated, she may unknowingly sabotage the maternal-infant bonding process during a subsequent pregnancy.

Most of the subsequent birth mothers we have known had not dealt adequately with their fears prior to their subsequent pregnancy. They were able to resolve most of the fears by simply confronting them. Some of these women were well into parenting their next child before finally coming to terms with their previous child's death. It is never too late to resolve unfinished business and bring past problems to a suitable ending.

What we call the beginning
is often the end.
And to make our ends
is to make a beginning
The end is where we start from.

T.S. Eliot

The Replacement Child

Do parents really try to replace one child with another as the term "replacement child" describes? Because of the unconscious need not to have to live with this intolerable pain of grief, some women do try to pretend that this terrible death didn't really happen by immediately wanting to get pregnant again and, as it were, to bear the same child that died. They quite often want a child of the same sex, and they want for the new child the name that was intended for the baby that died.

You may defend your desire to get pregnant immediately by saying "I am totally aware of my baby that died. I don't for a minute want to pretend that he never existed or that he can be replaced with another child. I just want a baby." Probably a more honest statement is that you want to be a mother. After physically and emotionally preparing yourself for these many months, you are eager for a child so that you can fulfill this role of mothering.

When you first thought about getting pregnant with the child that died, you had no strong attachment for *that* particular baby . . . you just wanted a baby. Any alive and healthy baby would satisfy your need. And most likely you still do want a baby. But because you did become attached during the pregnancy to the particular baby that died, you need to come to terms with the ending of that relationship, before you can want just any baby again. That's what the waiting is all about.

If your mother dies, people don't say "You can always have another mother." Then why is it all right to say you can always have another baby if your baby dies?

It's not just bereaved parents who fall into the "replacement child" trap. Friends, relatives and professionals are also likely to do the same thing. It's hard for them to appreciate the length of time it takes to readjust your life to that loss. Having another baby is a "quick fix" to that painful problem. Advising you to get pregnant right away to solve your problems is also a way for others to avoid having to think of your dead baby anymore. They mistakenly assume that your sad thoughts can be replaced with happy thoughts and then your grieving days are through.

It is inevitable that, from time to time, you will catch yourself getting your new child mixed up with the child that died. You can be sure that you will occasionally and inadvertently call him a her or vice versa. You may even find yourself calling your new baby by your dead baby's name. Parents of live children make that mistake, too. For that matter, you may even find yourself calling the child by the dog's name! These lapses are normal and not something to be overly concerned or self-conscious about.

The two main problems connected with having a "replacement child" are:

1. The parents delay their grief until after the new baby is born, or think they won't have to grieve at all if they have another baby soon. This then complicates the postpartum time with the new baby. These parents may find themselves unable to relate to this new child because the baby's arrival may open the unhealed wounds created by the previous child's death.

2. The subsequent child has an identity problem. This new child will be unable to be the "perfect" child that he is replacing, thus making it difficult for the parent to love this child as much as the dead baby.

Barbara's Story

Immediately following Holly's birth, I was lying in recovery trying to absorb what was happening. It all seemed too unreal at the time . . . very much like it was happening to someone else and I was just a third-party watching it all unfold. The pitocin was producing painful contractions and while everybody kept telling me it was o.k. to cry, I couldn't. It simply hurt too much. How unfair — I couldn't even cry. I was thinking about what was happening, that my daughter was dying, that I had a painful recovery period ahead just from the physical (not to mention emotional) stress, and it was all for **nothing.** When I voiced this feeling, my doctor cautioned me. He said that indeed Holly's life and death could be all for nothing if I thought it was. He pointed out that it was really up to me whether it was all for nothing or whether her life could be made to mean something.

I couldn't really comprehend what he was trying to say at the time. To me it just sounded like words. But with the passing of time it began to make sense. I began to see that Holly depended on me for her immortality — that as her mother I could make her life stand for something by growing from the experience. I realized that I could make her life touch others through my work. And so I began to take part in meaningful activities.

I had very strong feelings about the Baby Doe controversy that was in the news at the time and I decided to take action by writing a letter to the newspaper. It was wonderful therapy. I succeeded in getting a lot of anger out just in writing the letter. It helped me to get in touch with my own feelings about what had happened to Holly and also about the decisions we had made regarding her treatment. After the letter was published I received a lot of mail in support of what I said (and fortunately none in opposition). Some of the people who wrote expressed no feeling either way on the issue but simply wanted me to know that they were thinking about it. It made me feel good that something I had written might cause people to stop and rethink their views on this sensitive issue.

Later on, as I moved further down the road with my grief, I was able to reach out to others and listen as they talked about their loss. It gave me a good feeling to know that I might be lessening their load just by listening, but more than that, it gave me a better perspective on my own grief.

I could see that even though I still missed Holly, I wasn't hurting like I had during the first few months. I could see that I had once again begun to enjoy life and that I could smile and laugh now, something that at one time had seemed impossible. Most important of all though, I was helping someone else. I was able to help someone else to feel better because my daughter had lived . . . because my daughter had died. Through her short time with us she had caused something good to happen. This person had felt just a little better because I had listened, because I knew how she felt, because I had "been there." This was my goal: to make Holly's life stand for some positive change even after her death. I felt that if I could do something positive, then Holly's life was important and that her death had meaning. It was not all for nothing.

There were times during the early months following my loss when I cried out loud that I wished she had never been conceived. I felt that it would have been better for me if I had never experienced this pain. It was impossible for me to see anything positive in the whole experience. How fortunate that those days are over. I've gained so much from the experience. My capacity to feel joy has grown to greater heights because I've suffered the greatest loss of all and survived.

I also cherished the memories of my daughter's short life. From the beginning of the time I first felt movement, I could feel her feet very distinctly. We used to lie in bed at night and touch each other. It was almost like a game . . . I'd push her and she'd push back. We were touching in a way that only a mother can know and playing the only games we would ever play.

I'm left with two sons and I cherish their lives like nothing else. But I always wanted a daughter. There was a time when I agonized because I would never have one. Now I know that indeed, I did have one. She may have lived only a short time, but she was still my daughter. I'll never forget her. I never want to forget. She'll always be my baby girl. She will never break my heart. She will always be mine.

Barbara Stanbro

Chapter 2
Making Decisions About The Future

I don't ask for your pity, but just for your
　understanding
　　— not even that — no.
Just for the recognition of me in you,
　and the enemy time in us all.

Tennessee Williams

Who May See This "Next Pregnancy" as a Concern?

Even though a couple may want to have another baby, they may also be afraid of the pregnancy. What we've learned from talking with hundreds of couples is that those who have experienced one or more of the following usually will have more intense concerns about the subsequent or next pregnancy, than those who have not had such experiences.

— one or more spontaneous abortions or miscarriages
— the termination of a pregnancy
— a premature birth
— a stillbirth
— a neonatal death
— a birth of a handicapped child
— the release of a baby for adoption
— the loss of a child to sudden infant death syndrome
— the death of a child no matter what the age

What prompts this concern? Most often it is the simple realization that a second child could also die. What wasn't supposed to happen the first time did, so what's to stop it from happening again? Even where this particular fear is not acknowledged, a complicating factor may be the surfacing of unpleasant memories associated with the previous pregnancy. Instead of anticipating with enthusiasm the various stages of pregnancy the couple may be preoccupied with thoughts about what happened last time.

Another complicating factor that is present with some couples is guilt. The parents may wonder, "Will I be punished this time for some mistake I've made in my past?" "Will I be penalized because I had an abortion, or because I gave my first baby away?" Those who have not suffered the death or surrender of their own child may lightly remark that "lightning never strikes twice," or "you've paid your price." But couples who have been through the loss of a child are not easily convinced. They frequently see themselves as "marked" or singled out for repeated tragedy.

We know that in no way can we wipe away your past, nor do we assume that the information presented in this book will diminish your fears. We do hope, however, that what we have presented will better prepare you for what is to come and thus make the experience a more positive one.

Local Anesthetic

Sometimes
I think
That I'm not really present
At my life.
As though it goes on
Without my permission.

Sometimes,
Although I don't want to die,
I want to stop
Living.
I want to climb
Into the other side
Of my face
And observe my experiences
Without having them.

Sometimes,
And only once in a while,
I want to stop living.
But I really don't want
To die.

Merrit Malloy

"I'll never feel any better, so I might as well go ahead and get pregnant to make him happy."

"I am more afraid of being 60 with a 15 year old than forty with a newborn."

"It took me seven years to conceive the first time. To be told to wait a year before trying again made me feel desperate. I knew that waiting would add the risk of other problems."

"My biological clock continued to tick. The clock didn't stop just because I was grieving and was told to wait a year before trying again."

"If I could just get pregnant right away I could pretend this whole thing didn't happen."

"I just wanted a baby so I could be a happy person again."

"Everybody else wanted me to get pregnant again. I had no need to have another child. I felt that to do so would be a betrayal of my dead child. I have already used my love for that one. I felt it wouldn't be fair to have a child that I didn't really want. But was it fair for me to deprive the rest of the family?"

"Never again. The pain is unbearable. I won't set myself up only to have it happen again."

"It's just like falling off a horse. If I don't pick myself up and get back on that horse right away, I never will. It will be scary, I know, but much better when it's over."

When Should I Get Pregnant Again?

After reading the preceding pages you might suspect that we think you should wait as long as two years before even attempting another pregnancy. The truth is that we know of no ideal waiting period which will guarantee a subsequent pregnancy free of all the problems we have described.

Time is only as valuable as people make it. Time alone doesn't guarantee that things will be better later. One woman we knew moved to a new town soon after her baby died and never told anyone in the new community that she had borne a child. She and her husband rarely spoke about the baby to each other.Five years later she decided she wanted to have another baby, but the thought of going through the same thing again left her petrified. Because she needed to lose weight before getting pregnant (in preparation for surgery to correct a problem that could hinder future pregnancies) she used her weight as an excuse for avoiding pregnancy. As long as she didn't deal with the weight problem she didn't have to deal with her real fears about subsequent pregnancies. Those five years between her child's death and her deciding she wanted another baby counted for nothing. Those five years weren't used creatively to bring to completion that tragic part of her life. It then took her two more years of grief work before she felt ready to try again.

Another woman was ready to meet the challenge of another pregnancy only six months after her baby died. She had reconciled herself to her recent loss and was open to knowing that there were still some rocky times ahead for her. For her those six months were ones given to talking with others, reflecting, and searching for ways to come to terms with what had happened to her life.

Each person's history, emotional development, experience and support network is unique. All of these factors will help determine how quickly individuals will confront, and then work through, their grief.

Within two months after delivering a baby your body is usually physically able to carry another child. However there are potential psychological problems related to so hasty a pregnancy, beyond those we've described above. One is that your new baby's birth date will be very close to that of the baby that died, if the latter was full term.For several years your new baby's birthday may be clouded by sad memories of the baby that died. And if your earlier baby didn't live to be full term you may find yourself in the middle of a very intense grief time (your baby's actual due date) at a time when you are needing to concentrate on establishing a relationship with this new unborn child. Though at times this can't be prevented, it is something you will want to consider.

More importantly, however, we find that two months after the loss most parents are just beginning to work through the problems associated with bereavement. This tends to be a difficult time for bereaved parents because they are often no longer receiving emotional support from friends and relatives. They feel their life line has been cut. Many describe this time as one of disquieting tension.

We suggest that parents wait at least six months before

planning to conceive again. We don't assume that this will be an easy time for people, but we do believe it is an important time. Some people will be ready, some won't. And if you aren't ready, give yourself permission to wait a little longer.

How will you know for sure if you are ready to take the leap? Most likely you will feel good, and even at peace with the idea of being pregnant. Ask yourself these questions:

— How do I feel about holding other people's babies that are the same age that my child would have been?
— What do I think when I see other pregnant women?
— What will it be like for me to return to the same hospital where my dead baby was born?
— What is it like walking through the baby department at the store?

Your answer to these questions may help you to evaluate just how good you really are feeling about your new life. Do you turn away when you see a baby? Do you make every effort to avoid the baby department? Do you cry when you hear someone else had a baby? Can you see a difference between how you were feeling a month after your baby died and how you are feeling now? Do you have more control over when your tears will come? These are just clues that you still have some things to work out and that you may need some more time. Please don't assume that you have to be completely free of anger, resentment, or pain before planning another pregnancy. These questions are just offered as guidelines for you to use to help you confront some uncomfortable situations in your life so you can use your time effectively.

We are aware that many women will not take our advice and will say hello to another baby before saying a final good-bye to the one who has died. They too will survive the experience, even though the process will be more complicated. Again, waiting and even doing all you need to do to let go of your dead baby will not guarantee that you will not worry in the next pregnancy. But the possibility of your being able to look back and smile at yourself and lovingly take hold of your new baby will be better if you have given yourself sufficient transition time.

If I were to choose between pain and nothing I would choose pain.
William Faulkner

YES
   Is scary . . .

   It's so final
     So full
     So complete

NO
   Is easy . . .

   It closes doors
   And windows
   It hides facts
     and problems

No . . .
   Is an end.

But,
   YES . . .
   Is a beginning
   A pledge
     A promise
     A commitment . . .

Leonard Nimoy

Who Will Be Your Care Provider?

Who will be your care provider during your next pregnancy? Should you seek the services of the same professional who cared for you last time, or should you change? Your answers to the following questions will help you decide.

1. What level of care do I require for a safe outcome of this pregnancy based on my previous experience?
2. Will going to the care provider I had in the past be more or less comforting?
3. Will going to the same care provider require that I return to the same hospital, and is this a problem for me?
4. How will my partner feel about my choice?
5. Where will I feel most safe?

"Safe" is a relative term and requires defining in this situation. Of course you want to choose someone who is a competent practitioner in the field of obstetrics. A review of the circumstances surrounding your baby's death will help you determine whether or not you need a specialist. Equally important is your need for emotional support from your care provider. Because you will most likely feel emotionally vulnerable during this pregnancy you need someone with whom you can converse easily and frankly, with confidence that you are being heard and understood.

Remember that you are a consumer and that you can expect that your needs will be met (to the extent that this is actually possible) by your care provider. The other side of the coin is that you will need to trust your care provider with your feelings so he/she can respond to them.

A doctor may treat you as high risk if you have had a baby die, and introduce tests and procedures which are not generally necessary in a normal pregnancy. Some women, because of their fear of a repeat tragedy, will want this kind of care. Others will prefer to think of their pregnancy as normal and will want to assume that they will not have the extra tests and procedures associated with high risk, unless there is a definite clinical reason for them.

It is only fair to consider the needs of your care provider also. The purpose of taking an extensive history on a patient, along with a complete physical exam, is to be able to give complete, competent care. Your history, no matter what the cause of your baby's death, has a "red flag" on it. Even if everything is going fine, your doctor is more likely to be anxious about your pregnancy than he/she would be about the pregnancy of a woman who has not had a baby die. This is especially true if this doctor did not follow you during your last pregnancy or if there was no known cause for the baby's death. Your doctor wants you to be successful this time too and will want to take all the precautions necessary to help you accomplish your goal.

An important thing to remember is that you and your doctor will view this pregnancy differently. Your doctor has been involved with thousands of births and knows from experience and statistics that your chances for a healthy outcome are excellent. But because you have already been the loser in this lottery of life and death, you are not likely to be reassured by statistics. From your less objective point of view the chance of losing again is 100% no matter how the statistics read. You would love to believe your doctor when he says "It won't happen again," or "You let me do the worrying," or "Everything's fine," but it is highly unlikely that you will be able to do so. You might as well accept the truth that neither you nor the doctor will fully understand the other's viewpoint.

Things to think about

1. Don't assume your doctor knows how you are feeling. When asked, share how you are doing emotionally as well as physically. He or she won't know what's going on inside you unless you communicate.
2. Don't assume that the doctor is fully informed about your health history (especially if you haven't seen this doctor before). If you have been worried about fetal movements or some other symptom, make sure you feel satisfied with how the doctor deals with it. If you have a real concern it is unfair to your baby to play the "martyr role" by not speaking of your concern just because the doctor has not taken notice of it. Be assertive. You are a mother and have a child to look after.

Choices

As recently as 50 years ago the only alternative available to the childless couple was adoption. Today, however, the childless couple can choose from the buffet of options described below.

As you examine the options, you should ask yourself the following questions.

1. What is your reproductive history?
2. How important is it for you to be the biological parents of your children?
3. How much are you willing to spend? Many of the alternatives available to you are fairly expensive.
4. Do your religious beliefs limit the choices available to you?
5. How long are you willing to wait?
6. Are you willing to "play the odds"?
7. How strong are you when facing negative reactions from others around you?
8. Are both of you comfortable with the choice you've made?

The smorgasbord before you offers something for everyone, and new options are being researched every day. Knowing all the choices available to you allows you to make an informed decision. You will need to research them further to get more information.

1. **Attempting another pregnancy with your partner:** This is by far the easiest, and most acceptable to most people if the odds are in one's favor. You may need to confront your fears about your body failing you in the previous pregnancy and your concern that it will continue to betray you. Genetic and pre-pregnancy counseling can help to alleviate some fears through knowing your odds.

2. **Artificial insemination:** This procedure is used primarily by couples who learn through lab tests that the man's sperm count is either low or absent. If there is a genetically carried disorder in the couple, the use of donor sperm can eliminate the high odds of repeated tragedies in subsequent pregnancies. It can also be used to ensure a Rh-ve fetus for mothers with a high anti-D antibody level and a homozygous (for D antigen) partner. Statistically pregnancy occurs in 80% of cases within three months of monthly inseminations. Cost per insemination is approximately $100.00. This procedure is unacceptable to some due to ethical or cultural beliefs.

3. **Foster parenting:** For some couples this is the ideal choice. They have the opportunity to nurture and care for a child while still being able to place limitations on the time they are willing to give to the job. Some couples who have given birth to a child with a fatal illness can lovingly care for a foster child without the least bit of hesitation. Caring for a child of your own with limitations is a painful reminder to some that their

41

body failed them. Caring for a foster child with problems removes the personal identity crisis and just allows the parent to give love. Foster parenting can lead to adoption. Generally there is no cost to the family, and sometimes remuneration is provided for one's efforts.

4. **Adoption:** This is the most commonly talked about alternative for the childless couple. There are disputes as to whether adoption is accessible to most people due to a baby shortage. Others will claim that if parents pursue and do not limit themselves on what child is acceptable to them they will indeed find a child. Frustrations and anxieties run high in families waiting to adopt. The cost of adoption depends on whether you are dealing with a private professional person (usually lawyer or doctor) or adoption agency, the latter being less costly as a rule.

5. **Surrogate mothering:** This is a relatively new, and somewhat controversial way to resolve the problem of the mother's infertility. The sperm of the father is artificially inseminated into a donor mother. After delivery the baby is adopted. Surrogate mothering assures that at least the father is biologically connected to the child. The adopting couple do have the opportunity to specify ethnic background, education, etc. of the surrogate mother. This option is not legal in most states to date and it can be costly depending on the fees charged by the surrogate mother, and by the attorney who makes the legal arrangements.

6. **Choosing a childfree marriage:** After looking at all the options you may decide it's okay not to be parents after all. Childfree living is different from being childless. Being childless presents the image of this unhappy, possibly bitter couple coping with their misfortune. Deciding to be childfree is not just a different word to make something tragic digestible. Rather, childfree means the couple has made a positive step in getting on with the rest of their lives together. They can indeed have full and rewarding lives even without children in their home.

**The gods have two ways
of dealing harshly with us.
The first is to deny us our
dreams, and the second is
to grant them.**

Oscar Wilde

Adoption

Pregnancy, labor, delivery and parenting present obvious anxious moments for bereaved parents going through a subsequent pregnancy. So does choosing to adopt a child. People sometimes assume that arranging for an adoption frees one from the endless hours of worry associated with a subsequent pregnancy. Not so. Adoption may have its advantages, but freedom from anxiety is not one of them.

Friends and relatives may encourage you to consider adoption rather than taking a risk of having another disappointing pregnancy outcome. For them the "best way" and least risk involved for you to achieve your family may seem very obvious. Remember, it is always easier to look at someone else's dilemmas and find solutions to their problems. You may also find that your dead baby will no longer be significant in their minds once you've started adoption procedures. It's the same withdrawal of grief support that bereaved parents going through a subsequent pregnancy experience. A new positive direction is supposed to restore your previous optimistic thinking. It's just not that easy. You may need to gently remind your well-meaning friends that this new child is not meant to take the place of your child that died and what you need from them is patience and compassion.

The decision to adopt is not a simple one. Feelings of failure or the idea that adopting is second best have to be wrestled with and resolved before finally deciding that adoption is a good way to increase your family. For some women the experience of pregnancy itself is important, as is having a child who is "of my own flesh." Other women couldn't care less about these considerations. It is important to know your own mind and to resolve these issues at the outset, because any unresolved feelings will affect how you relate to your adopted child. You may find that when you finally get down to just wanting to be parents all of these other issues will tend to melt away.

Everything we have said about timing the start of a subsequent pregnancy applies as well to the timing of an adoption. Waiting for an adoption to come through is similar to waiting for your pregnancy to come to full term. The anticipation and planning and mental preparation for this adopted child needs to happen, but if you are still actively mourning your baby's death the bonding to this new child will be delayed.

Not all adoption arrangements work out as planned. The birth mother may change her mind and decide not to relinquish the infant even after you've prepared yourself for this

43

new child. Though this rarely occurs (1% to 2% of the time, the same rate as for neonatal death) you need but one clear example to remind you that it could happen to you. If it does happen the grief you will experience will be similar to the grief that you felt after your baby died. Even after you have taken the child into your home, you may find it difficult to believe that this new treasure won't also be taken from you. During the probationary period of three to six months after the initial adoption you may be beset with fears that the baby will be snatched from you. Because of these fears you may find yourself putting up a protective emotional shield to guard you from being hurt again. This response is quite normal and natural but it needs to be recognized and dealt with.

Subsequent adoptive parents are not less apprehensive and protective about their baby's safety than are those parents who were pregnant with a subsequent child. Adoptive parents acknowledge that they too frequently and compulsively check on their babies to reassure themselves that these little ones are alive and well. The mere fact that the baby is not born by you does not protect you from the fear that something could happen to this child as well.

Every state has its own rules concerning adoptions. Private and agency adoptions have different guidelines and you should learn all you can about these before making a decision about which way to go. Infants will be less available than older children. The less you limit your specifications as to age, race, and other differences, the easier it will be for a child to be placed in your care.

Peggy's Story

Our daughter Micalee was stillborn on September 2, 1981. She had been the answer to a prayer, after six years of infertility. We had been through the infertility workup; minor surgery and drugs had helped us achieve the long awaited pregnancy. Now, after nine months of joy in anticipation, we were not only back to being childless. Now we were also bereaved parents.

The first month of our grief was terrible. Since I was already 33 years old, we already had plans to wait six months and "try again," assuming that our infertility problem had been solved and that we had the option of another preg-

nancy. The autopsy report changed all that. We were told that although Micalee had died of a cord accident — a cause of death that was unlikely to be repeated — she also had a rare fatal disease which would have ended her life by the age of ten. The worst news was that the disease might be genetic, with a 25% chance that any subsequent biological child would also die young. We felt we could not take the chance of risking the death of another child. This meant that we had lost not only Micalee but also any future opportunity to bear children. Our grief doubled and redoubled. We were grieving over the loss of many children.

Six weeks after Micalee's death we attended our first meeting of The Compassionate Friends and also joined Resolve, a support group for infertile couples. It was important for us to have both groups. Members of Compassionate Friends were able to understand our grief over Micalee's death, though it was hard for them to relate to our infertility. Resolve was a great resource for information about infertility, but its members understood little about the loss of Micalee.

Shortly thereafter a friend suggested the possibility of Artificial Insemination by Donor (AID). We would thus have the shared experience of another pregnancy, the child would be half ours genetically, and we would be avoiding the 25% risk of a fatal disease. It all sounded so simple. During months two and three after Micalee's death we carefully avoided an accidental pregnancy while taking my temperature daily in order to have charts to show the doctors as part of the AID program. In January, four months into the grief process, we began the program.

The AID program added considerable stress to our lives. At first our strong desire for conception enabled us to cope with the dehumanizing aspects of AID. We became familiar with the process that we would have to repeat on each of the days which the doctors had determined would be ideal for conception: First I would go to the doctor's office to have my mucus checked. Then after getting dressed, going to another location to get a sperm sample, and yet another place to pay for it, I would go back to the doctor's office, undress again so that I could be inseminated by a nurse. Finally, after lying on my back for fifteen minutes crying "I want Micalee," I would get dressed again and pay for the nurse's "services." This process was repeated on two or three separate days during midcycle.

45

After six years of timing our lovemaking by the thermome-ter in order to become pregnant, it was just too emotion-ally draining carefully to avoid pregnancy at home, while at the same time trying to achieve pregnancy at a "service station" for insemination. We'd had enough, so we quit the program.

We made application for adoption through an agency and also got a lead on a possible private adoption. The due date for this latter baby was just before Christmas. A few days before the due date we went out for dinner and one last time alone together. During dinner I started crying, and said, "I don't want this baby. I want Micalee!" I was surprised at my words and the strength of my feelings. I thought I had let go of her, but obviously this was not the case.

On Christmas Day we were told that the biological mother had decided not to release her baby for adoption. Once more we were childless with no remedy in sight. The agency called us in January about a biracial baby due at the end of the month. Because no one else had indicated an interest in biracial children, we found ourselves suddenly at the top of the waiting list. Again we went out to dinner; again I cried for Micalee; and again the birth mother cancelled the adop-tion.

Sometime in February, eighteen months after Micalee's death and after several unsuccessful AID and adoption at-tempts, we came to the point where at last we let go of our daughter and accepted the fact that we might remain child-less. We decided that if I didn't become pregnant within another three and a half years (after 10 years of trying), we would quit trying and get on with our life without children. I finally felt some peace in spite of my infertility and the loss of our daughter.

On March 10, through an adoption agency, we met a 22-month-old boy who soon became our son. In the days be-fore he came to our home there were no tears or "I want Micalee" thoughts. When Isaiah did arrive at our home we were ready for him. It is fortunate that those other babies had not become ours. They would have had to compete with Micalee. As it worked out we are able to give Isaiah our undivided love.

Peggy Swanton

Chapter 3
Medical Considerations

The decision to conceive again after a lost pregnancy may or may not be influenced by an understanding of the causes of the loss or an appreciation of how the past events may affect the future pregnancy. Ideally the pregnancy will be a planned event, ideal in the sense that the planning will involve an analysis of the past and a determination to take the necessary steps to avoid a recurrence when — and this is by no means always the case — particular factors can be identified.

Though there were some early attempts to study the causes of stillbirth and neonatal death, it was not until the middle of this century that an appreciation of the causes began to evolve. Epidemiological studies showed that there were major international and regional differences and that the most important influences were sociological rather than purely "medical." The poorest outcomes were in groups disadvantaged by poverty and its attendant inadequate nutrition, hygiene, and housing, along with a tendency toward repeated pregnancies and susceptibility to infectious disease. Perinatal mortality rates, including stillbirth and early neonatal deaths, are one of the indices by which pregnancy outcome is judged. These rates have shown a steady fall in the last three decades, the rate in the United States now being little more than 1 in 100.

When detailed analyses of deaths were first made the causes were identified in three main groups: prematurity, asphyxia, and congenital abnormality. Included in the category of prematurity were babies who were mature but poorly grown and therefore of low birth weight, but mistakenly assumed to be premature. Included in the asphyxia group were babies who had suffered trauma during the process of birth.

The three main groups still exist, though prematurity now accounts for two thirds of the deaths, and asphyxia during labor and birth trauma have been greatly reduced.

There have been a number of important advances during the last two decades. These include the following: improvement in the care of low birth weight infants, understanding of the relationship between early and adequate prenatal care and outcome, technological advances, such as ultrasound and fetal monitoring, that allow for observation of the fetus before birth; introduction of prophylaxis against rhesus sensitization; avoidance of birth trauma; recognition that exposure of the mother to some drugs, infections, and environmental hazards also leads to exposure of the fetus; and better control of diabetes in the pregnant woman.

This is some of the good news. The darker side of the picture is that though more premature babies survive, there has been little improvement in the rate of premature births; the causes of many lethal abnormalities are still not understood; many women still do not have easy access to prenatal care; and deaths — particularly stillbirths — still occur where there is "no explanation." More importantly, for parents who have suffered a loss, the perinatal mortality rate is still much too high. These parents will gain limited consolation from the observation that the perinatal mortality rate is now half what it was two decades ago.

Risk identification is now an essential part of prenatal care. Any system will include the history of a stillbirth or neonatal death as a major risk factor, and the pregnancy of a person with this history is likely to be identified as high risk. In a generalization that includes a spectrum ranging from those who have no increased risk of a recurrence to those who have a considerable risk, one's place on the spectrum can only be determined by a study of individual circumstances. Such a study requires a review of the past medical history, previous successful obstetric history, current medical status, and the details of the unsuccessful pregnancy.

In recent years there has been an important development in the effort to minimize pregnancy loss — the concept of preconception counseling. In preconception counseling a couple explores with the counselor the actual risk involved in a planned pregnancy. Often the evaluation reveals minimal risk with no need for preconception intervention, but in some situations careful planning with appropriate intervention will be indicated. Previous pregnancy loss is one of these situations.

The preconception evaluation has two parts: (1) an assessment of those physical factors that may or may not increase the risk of recurrence and a consideration of how they might be influenced, and (2) a feel for the emotional burden involved in another pregnancy, followed by the development of a strategy for emotional support during and after the pregnancy.

One of the great frustrations surrounding any pregnancy loss is the potential for uncertainty — the lack of any clear understanding of "what went wrong" — a frustration sometimes compounded by a reluctance to carefully investigate the clinical circumstances involved in the death in a mistaken attempt to resolve the emotional pain as quickly as possible. Often glib assurances are offered to reassure the family (e.g. "lightning never strikes twice in the same place"), but these assurances are usually based on a genuine desire to ease the pain rather

49

than on any objective and scientific assessment of the facts. The issue is relatively simple. Will it happen again? How can we prevent it from happening again?

The starting point for preconception counseling in this context is obvious. Was there a clear pathological diagnosis to account for the complications that led to the baby's death or was there not? Where there was a clear diagnosis then there is *always* a statistical basis on which to forecast the likelihood of a recurrence and there is *always* an opportunity to review options for intervention that may alter that risk. Even when there is no pathologic diagnosis there is usually a statistical basis on which to forecast the risk of recurrence. These statistics are available and should be sought. Of course there is little consolation in recognizing that even if something as rare as 1:2000 has happened to you already, the risk of it happening again are still 1:2000. Nevertheless understanding of risk, based on statistics, is the only basis for the rational management of the next pregnancy.

Basic Questions that will help gather information

1. At what stage of pregnancy did delivery or death before delivery occur?
2. Did the baby show evidence of congenital anomaly?
3. Is there a family history of a similar occurrence?
4. Was there evidence of maternal illness? If so, did it precede the pregnancy or did it only develop during the pregnancy?
5. Was an autopsy and placental examination performed?
6. Was a Chromosomal analysis prepared?
7. Was a cause (a) clearly identified? (b) suggested but not confirmed? (c) not identified?
8. Had the baby achieved a weight appropriate for its gestational age?
9. Was there any evidence of external influences such as medications, alcohol, etc. that could have been factors?

The time flow charts below and the list of questions above are a simplified outline of a system for reviewing the previous pregnancy. The process must involve the obtaining of all the old medical records with two purposes in mind: (1) an analysis of the risk of recurrence and (2) an identification of those steps that can be taken to reduce the risk. A strategy for risk reduction should be established and then additional steps identified that would be taken solely to provide support and reassurance for the mother and family during the pregnancy. This strategy can only be developed after the risks have been identified and medically necessary interventions planned. It has to be emphasized that there are no absolute recommendations for additional support and there is a tremendous variation in the needs of families. Some families need continuous demonstration that all is well. Others are either confident anyway or feel that more detailed investigation will only increase, rather than decrease, their anxiety.

As the strategy is developed various emphases can be applied to the time frame of the pregnancy. These are presented below with the qualification that all care needs to be individualized.

Preconception
Emotional preparation
Nutritional review
Assessment of maternal health
Control of chronic disease, diabetes, hypertension, etc.
Optimizing drug regimes — least effective dose
Correcting uterine anomalies
Rubella immunity

First Trimester
(Conception to three months)
Early confirmation of intrauterine pregnancy
Standard prenatal laboratory testing
Avoidance of teratogens
* Chorionic villus biopsy in some high recurrence risk conditions
Accurate dating — ultrasound, if necessary
Confirmation of heart tones — usually at ten weeks
* Screenings for some infectious agents

Second Trimester
(three to six months)
* Amniocentesis, when indicated; prenatal diagnosis and alpha fetoprotein screening
Routine care with emphasis on fetal growth
* Cervical cerclage
* 20 to 24 Week amniocentesis for rhesus (other) Sensitization
* Bed rest
* Prophylactic tocolysis
* Screening for some infectious agents
Glucose tolerance screen
* Ultrasound for anomalies

51

Third Trimester

(Six months to term)

Routine care with emphasis on fetal growth, position,
    condition and maternal health

Childbirth preparation classes

* Ultrasound, fetal growth, placenta localization, anomalies

Fetal movement counts

* Biophysical profiles

* Plans for delivery: vaginal or cesarean

                        spontaneous onset vs. induced

                        selection of anesthesia

Screening for infectious agents

Newborn care

*Only required when specifically indicated

Common Reasons Why Babies Die

It is not possible to list every cause of perinatal death. What follows is a list of the more common causes, a brief explanation of how the condition causes a death, and an estimate of the likelihood of a recurrence. It has to be emphasized that statistics can be very misleading. Although we have a good idea of the incidence of any given condition in pregnancy, there is still a tremendous individual variation and it is very difficult to give an actual figure for the chances of a death occurring in a particular clinical condition, for the simple reason that once the condition is recognized, appropriate steps can be taken to prevent the death from occurring.

Some conditions such as diabetes exist as a constant theme throughout an individual's pregnancy. Others, such as cord prolapse, occur as a single event. Still others occur as an apparently random event the first time, but, having occurred once, are more likely to occur again in a subsequent pregnancy. Placental abruption is an example of this latter category.

Statistics should be used objectively to provide an overall understanding of the natural history of any given condition, but statistics can be misleading and can be used in different ways. For example, a 5% chance of a recurrence in a condition that only occurs 1 in every 100 times represents a five-fold increase in risk. But to say that the risk of recurrence has increased five-fold sounds very different from saying that there is a 95% chance that the particular event will not occur again! Therefore, statistics have to be used with caution and with appropriate and careful individualization.

52

Asphyxia

With the advances in modern obstetric care, it is quite unusual for a baby to die during the course of labor or delivery. Just one or two generations ago this was not so. We can thank modern technology for making childbirth safer. Asphyxia, for example, has been sharply reduced by ultrasound and monitoring of fetal blood samples. Current obstetric practice also appreciates that the fetus is not just a passive participant in the process.

Strictly speaking, asphyxia is an imprecise term. It represents all the changes that occur when the baby is deprived of oxygen. In anoxia, oxygen is absent, in hypoxia it is reduced below normal needs.

Asphyxia can occur in the following situations:

Maternal illness: The mother's blood is low in oxygen.

Placental Insufficiency: The placenta does not pass oxygen across to the baby's blood. This condition can arise from the illness of the mother, or because of an excessively long pregnancy.

Increased uterine pressure: The uterine contractions may be too strong or too frequent and obstruct the circulation in the placenta.

Placental abruption: The placenta may separate from the uterus prematurely, so that oxygen won't pass well to the baby, before delivery.

Cord obstruction: The umbilical cord protrudes through the cervix, or fetal parts press on the cord thus decreasing the oxygen supply to the baby.

Most instances of hypoxia during labor don't actually cause the death of the baby, but produce warning signals such as abnormal heart rates, or passage of dark green-stained fluid from the uterus, known as meconium, the baby's first stool. These signs are defined as FETAL DISTRESS and should lead to individual evaluation, treatment, and if indicated, delivery by cesarean section or forceps. Some of the deaths that occur before labor and particularly those occurring unexpectedly between 20 and 30 weeks, may be due to "asphyxia." That information alone is not an adequate explanation. The physician should try to identify the problems that led to the asphyxia.

Abruption

Abruption, or the separation of the placenta from the wall of the uterus before the onset of labor, is a potentially serious complication of pregnancy. The separation may occur spontaneously or it may occur in association with maternal illness, particularly hypertension. The abruption may be partial or complete, and may cause severe disturbances to the mother's blood coagulation system. The more severe the abruption, the more likely it is that the fetus will become hypoxic.

Abruption tends to recur in at least 15% of previous cases. It is also important to know that cocaine or amphetamine use in pregnancy is likely to cause abruption.

Intrauterine Growth Retardation

Truly chronic hypoxia is most likely to be reflected in a condition known an intrauterine growth retardation, where the absence of oxygen and other nutrients over a long period of time may have affected the baby's growth so that the baby is small for its gestational age. These babies do not withstand the stress of labor as well as fully grown babies, and signs of distress are likely to occur during the course of labor. Intrauterine growth retardation is not only caused by poor placental function with or without maternal illness. When there is a nutritional or respiratory type of growth retardation, then there is an asymmetry to the baby's growth. The head grows at a relatively normal rate with the rest of the body lagging behind. When the baby is growing poorly because of a problem within itself, rather than in the placenta, such as in some types of congenital anomaly or a congenitally acquired infection, then the lack of growth is spread out more evenly and the baby is symmetrically small. Other conditions that can be associated with intrauterine growth retardation include chronic heart disease, severe anemia, severe asthma, or conditions where there is pre-existing damage to the mother's circulatory system, such as in some advanced cases of diabetes.

Diabetes

Intrauterine growth retardation can occur in association with diabetes, but the more commonly recognized problem with diabetes is excessive growth of the baby. Tremendous progress has been made in understanding the problem of diabetes in pregnancy and now the prospects of diabetic mothers are little worse than for other women. The key to the management of the diabetic pregnancy is rigorous control of the blood sugar levels. This should start even before conception occurs and the blood sugar should be maintained in a very normal range — 80 to 100 milligrams percent throughout the pregnancy. When this is done there is no increase in congenital anomaly, no increase in stillbirth, no increase in overweight babies and no increase in problems of immaturity associated with diabetes. In the past all of these conditions have contributed to outcomes that were three or four times worse in diabetic pregnancies than in normal pregnancies, but the outcome these days is very much better as long as tight control is applied.

Multiple Pregnancy

Twin pregnancy occurs in approximately 1% of patients, and other multiple pregnancies — triplets, etc. — much less frequently. The fertility drugs that are now widely used increase the incidence of multiple pregnancy over the natural rate. Twin pregnancy can arise from the fertilization of two separate eggs (dizygotic twins) or from the fertilization of a single egg which splits into two pregnancies (monozygotic twins). Twin pregnancies are at greater risk of premature labor, of difficulties in delivery because of abnormal positioning of the babies, and of certain medical complications of pregnancy such as hypertension, and the development of excess amniotic fluid (polyhydramnios). There is further risk when the fetuses share a single placenta or occupy the same amniotic sac; when a complication known as twin transfusion syndrome occurs, where one fetus develops at the expense of the other; or when there is cord entanglement between the twins.

There are a number of influences that affect the likelihood of twin pregnancy, in addition to the fertility drugs already mentioned. Monozygotic twinning is much more common with advancing maternal age, whereas in dizygotic twinning racial differences are a factor. Europeans are more likely to have twins than Japanese, for example. Familial inculdence is also important. There is a higher incidence of twins in female relatives of women who have themselves born dizygotic twins.

In the past twin pregnancy often went undiagnosed until late in the pregnancy or even during labor. Now, with the availability of ultrasound, earlier diagnosis is typical and multiple pregnancies can be more closely watched.

Obviously, nothing can be done to alter the situation when a placenta or sac is shared. Unfortunately there has been only limited success in preventing premature labor, even with complete bed rest and other treatments. The improvement of the outcome of twin pregnancy is more likely to come from careful surveillance and timing of early delivery in those pregnancies where one or both of the twins is "getting into trouble."

Preterm Delivery

The single most important cause of perinatal loss is immaturity. Even though the perinatal death rate has been greatly reduced in the last twenty years, there has been little reduction in the rate of premature births. It is true that there have been excellent advances in neonatal care, so that many more babies are surviving. Most, but not all are surviving without disabilities. Still, one of the goals of prenatal care is to prevent premature birth. Although excellent prenatal care has been shown to be effective in reducing the incidence of premature births, premature deliveries still occur. Many women, for a variety of reasons, are receiving inadequate prenatal care, thus greatly increasing their risks of premature delivery.

Some early deliveries occur spontaneously as a result of obvious complications of pregnancy. Some of them occur as a result of obstetric interventions to help the mother, e.g. in severe pregnancy induced hypertension, and some of them occur for no apparent reason. It is difficult to generalize about the chances of a premature delivery occurring in any subsequent pregnancy. When the delivery has been the result of the premature onset of contractions or early rupture of the membranes, the cause is sometimes an abnormality in the uterus such as fibroids or the presence of a septum, or an abnormality in the cervix such as a condition known as "incompetent cervix." X-ray of the uterus — hysterography or inspection of the uterine cavity — hysteroscopy, can be undertaken between pregnancies to check for these defects and to permit remedial action.

Some premature deliveries occur in association with multiple pregnancy or with acute complications of pregnancy such as placental abruption or acute polyhydramnios. There is a strong probability that infection may be responsible when no other cause is evident.

Infection

Historically, there has been a fear of infection during labor and delivery. Childbirth fever used to occur in epidemic proportion prior to a clearer understanding of the natural history of infection and the later availability of antibiotics. The focus of the risk of infection has now been turned away from the mother and greater attention is currently given to the ever present threat to the baby. The premature infant in particular is less able to withstand bacterial infection acquired at the time of delivery, and as noted above there is increasing evidence that infection that has been dormant in the mother may be the cause for some of the otherwise unexplainable premature labors.

Infection can be acquired by the fetus during pregnancy as a result of transmission through the placenta, such as with rubella or cytomegalic virus, syphilis, or it can be acquired by the infant during delivery such as with herpes, hepatitis or beta hemolytic streptococcus. Very few infections recur in subsequent pregnancies. Infections that occur coincidentally during pregnancy and then are transmitted through the placental circulation to the baby, are unlikely to recur in subsequent pregnancies because by then the mother has acquired immunity. Infections that are truly chronic or recurrent, such as herpes, can usually be identified ahead of time and necessary precautions taken to improve the safety of delivery.

A major problem with understanding the relationship between infection and premature rupture of the membranes or premature labor stems from the fact that certain bacteria are normally present in the vagina and, for the most part, cause no harm. However, some of these bacteria may be responsible for causing infection in the fetus once the membranes have ruptured, and others not normally present in the vagina may be responsible for the initiation of early labor or for causing early rupture of the membranes.

Congenital Anomaly

Approximately 3% of all newborn infants will have some form of congenital anomaly. These anomalies range from relatively tiny imperfections to major structural defects that are incompatible with survival. The development of these defects may be predetermined by chromosomal abnormality or they may develop during the course of organ and system formation in the first three months of pregnancy. The causes of many of these abnormalities are not well understood. Some may be due to relatively slight problems with blood supply at a critical stage of development. Others may be due to toxic environment effects, such as occurred with the prescription of Thalidomide.

The crucial response to a congenital anomaly is to make a specific diagnosis based, where possible and where relevant, on a chromosomal analysis, and to research the well documented facts surrounding the chances of recurrence. These chances may vary between a no greater than average chance of a rare random occurrence to a 50% chance of a recurrence of a "dominant" defect.

Erythroblastosis Fetalis

One of the major success stories in the field of preventive medicine in the last generation has been the application of anti-D gamma globulin prophylaxis programs for rhesus negative mothers. As a result of these programs there has been a significant reduction in the incidence of rhesus isoimmunization and the consequent effects on the fetus. Severely affected babies used to develop extensive edema, a condition described as hydrops fetalis. Hydrops fetalis still occurs, but much less frequently, and rhesus incompatibility is now one of the least common causes of this condition. More likely causes of hydrops fetalis include sensitivity to other antibodies, congenital cardiac disease in the infant, metabolic disorders and certain other abnormalities. Again, when there is a past history of hydrops fetalis an expert should be consulted to determine whether there is any chance of a recurrence in a subsequent pregnancy.

Unexplained Stillbirth

With the increased attention to the fetus during the course of labor, a sudden death of the baby during labor is a relatively rare occurrence. Occasionally (about one in 500 pregnancies) there is an acute complication with the cord (cord prolapse). This condition is most likely to occur when the maternal pelvis is not occupied by the baby's head during the early part of labor. Stillbirths usually happen unexpectedly during the course of pregnancy, before the onset of labor, and this is one area where modern obstetrics has not had a major impact. It is likely that a significant number of these otherwise unexplained stillbirths are associated with genetic abnormalities and, where possible, tissue should have been obtained from either the fetus or the membranes at the time of delivery. This is especially important when the baby shows external signs of abnormality. Other possible causes of unexplained stillbirth before labor include intrauterine infection and blood transfusion between the fetus and the mother.

Multiple Spontaneous Abortions

Miscarriages, or spontaneous abortions are relatively common in a woman's reproductive history. As many as 20% of all recognized conceptions end in spontaneous abortion, the majority of these losses being in the first trimester. Because of our recent ability to diagnose pregnancy quite early women are now more aware of their early pregnancy losses. In the past an early miscarriage may have just been viewed as a late or unusually heavy period.

Chromosomal anomalies make up a large percentage of these early pregnancy losses. Most chromosomal anomalies are considered random events and do not necessarily repeat themselves. A medical approach to accepting these early losses as the body's natural defense against developing abnormal offspring is logical, but less than comforting to the hopeful parent. Though the hardship of caring for a severely handicapped child is obvious, a strictly medical approach to miscarriage denies the expectant parent's need for emotional support.

Mid-trimester losses tend to involve genetically normal fetuses. This fact leads medical investigators to suspect infection or a disturbance in the maternal immunologic system or a structural defect in the uterus or cervix to be the cause of many of these pregnancy losses. Treating these particular problems in individual cases seems to diminish recurrence.

The woman who experiences multiple spontaneous abortions (3 or more consecutive losses) can now view her future with more hope than was once assumed. In spite of the experience of 2, 3, or more previous miscarriages most women, with appropriate care will have a 75% chance of a successful pregnancy. For practical and economic reasons most physicians do not recommend extensive testing until after the third loss. A careful review of her general health, infection screening, checking for structural abnormalities of her reproductive system and immunological studies may uncover correctable problems.

Summary

The above review is by no means comprehensive. It is intended to provide a simple explanation of some complex events that can have major impact. It is intended to encourage a systematic review of the events of the previous pregnancy so that plans for management of the subsequent pregnancy can be placed in a true and realistic perspective. It is important to obtain old records and to review them in detail. At first glance such records may not appear to include much useful information, but often some careful sleuthing can uncover facts that will be very helpful during the next pregnancy.

Prenatal Diagnostic Tests That Help Determine Fetal Health and Well Being

Special Tests

There is now almost daily progress in our understanding of the genetic basis for many diseases and in our ability to diagnose these diseases prenatally. It is most important, whenever personal or family history includes the diagnosis of a disease for which there is a known hereditary basis, that counseling is obtained from a genetic counselor who is in touch with the rapidly expanding information that is becoming available in that specialty. On occasion, this may lead to a referral to a regional center.

Alpha Fetoprotein

Alpha fetoprotein is a major component of fetal blood. Small amounts of AFP are found in the amniotic fluid of normal fetuses as well as in the maternal serum. In the presence of a neural tube defect, abdominal wall imperfection or other malformations, concentrations of AFP in the amniotic fluid and maternal serum are increased. Low levels of AFP are in some cases associated with chromosomal anomalies. The most precise prediction of the likelihood of a chromosomal anomaly can be made by correlating the AFP levels with the age of the mother. Once a statistical probability is identified, a decision can be made as to whether amniocentesis or chorionic villus biopsy is required. It is important to date the pregnancy accurately when alpha fetoprotein is used, since the levels vary according to gestational age.

Ultrasound exam will date the pregnancy with reasonable accuracy, and will identify multiple pregnancies (associated with high levels of AFP). It will also demonstrate most body malformations.

Chromosomal Analysis

Analysis of the chromosomal make-up of the fetal cells (genotype) can be performed on cells obtained from the amniotic fluid by amniocentesis. Ideally this procedure takes place between 14 and 16 weeks after the pregnancy begins.

A good alternative to **amniocentesis** is **chorionic villus biopsy.** The advantage of this technique is that it is done much earlier in pregnancy. The results are available within a few days, so that a decision as to whether to terminate the pregnancy or not can be made by the end of the first trimester. When the technique was first being developed, there were concerns that

60

there would be an increased risk of infection and subsequent miscarriage. These initial fears have not been borne out, and chorionic villus biopsy is increasingly replacing amniocentesis for prenatal diagnosis.

Amniotic Fluid Studies

Amniotic fluid in the later two thirds of the pregnancy is derived almost exclusively from the fetal urine. Analysis of the amniotic fluid can therefore provide important information about the degree of hemolysis (blood breakdown) when there is rhesus or other blood group isoimmunization. The blood is broken down into bilirubin which is then excreted through the kidneys into the amniotic sac.

Later in the pregnancy an analysis of the amniotic fluid will reveal the degree of maturity of the baby's lungs. The fatty substances that help to maintain expansion of the baby's lungs when the baby takes its first breath are also excreted into the amniotic fluid where they can be measured to provide an accurate prediction of the likelihood of respiratory difficulties during the newborn period. Testing of the amniotic fluid is particularly important when delivery is anticipated before thirty-four weeks gestation.

Not only does the amniotic fluid contain fetal urine, but on occasion it also contains fetal bowel contents. Most often the presence of bowel contents (meconium) in the amniotic fluid is not very important, particularly if there is a good volume of amniotic fluid. This is a detail that should be noted in labor, however, and special precautions should be taken to monitor the condition of the fetus and to ensure that the baby does not inhale the thick meconium material into the lungs at the time of delivery. The incidental discovery of meconium when amniocentesis is performed in the second trimester of pregnancy is probably of no great importance as long as the other investigations, such as ultrasound, do not show any abnormality.

Ultrasound

Part of the revolution in obstetric care in the past 10 to 15 years has been due to the availability and increasing sophistication in the ultrasound imaging of the fetus inside the uterus. Ultrasound, which utilizes high frequency sound waves to construct an image of the fetus, started with static, "still life" imaging. Since then more dynamic, "cinematic" imaging techniques have been developed.

Ultrasound can be used as early as the sixth week to demonstrate the normal location of the fetus in the uterus, to rule out ectopic pregnancy and to help in the assessment of bleeding in early pregnancy where miscarriage might be a possibility.

Early measurement of the pregnancy sac helps with accurate dating as does measurement of the actual size of the fetus throughout pregnancy. However, as one would anticipate, the measurement of the size becomes less accurate as pregnancy advances and individual variations in size become more obvious.

In the second part of pregnancy, ultrasound is used for helping with amniocentesis, for demonstrating normal or abnormal fetal structure, for localizing of the placenta, and for confirming the presence of multiple pregnancy.

ANTENATAL FETAL MONITORING

Ultrasound is often used in a serial fashion. This is particularly important when the fetus is being monitored for growth patterns, and serial measurements are required to demonstrate normal or abnormal growth. Such is the case in intrauterine growth retardation which may appear on its own or in association with hypertensive disease of pregnancy or in the management of diabetic pregnancies where excessive fetal growth may be a problem.

Antenatal Biophysical Profile

At the end of the pregnancy, ultrasound can be used to assess fetal function by looking at fetal movements and muscle tone using a technique described as biophysical profile. This technique also uses measurement of the volume of the amniotic fluid to assess the well-being of the fetus. It has been recognized that when there is an acute reduction in the volume of amniotic fluid this could indicate an acute deterioration in the baby's health and therefore a reduction in urine output. The reduction in amniotic fluid may also be associated with abnormalities involving the kidney, and ultrasound is used to identify kidney and bladder structure as well as function. Similarly, an excessive amount of amniotic fluid sometimes may be associated with a fetal anomaly, and careful ultrasound can help to identify or rule out abnormalities when there is an excess of fluid.

Antenatal Fetal Heart Rate Monitoring

Another means of assessing the baby's response to its environment is to monitor the fetal heart rate. The baby is considered to be healthy when its heart rate increases temporarily in response to movements, producing a "reactive" trace. An even more sensitive test involves checking the heart rate in response to contractions. This technique usually involves stimulating the nipple to release sufficient hormones to cause contractions, but not enough to initiate labor. In a pregnancy where the baby is in good condition and there is good "placental reserve" then there are no alterations in the heart rate in association with the contractions. When there is a relative reduction in oxygenation to the fetus, then there may be a slowing of the heart rate after the contraction has occurred.

Fetal Movement Counts

An even more accessible, and certainly economical, test of fetal condition is the measurement of the movements that the fetus makes during a given time period at various times during the day. It has been observed that a significant reduction in movements may be related to a deterioration of the baby's condition. Many mothers find that they can get in tune with their babies by devoting thirty to sixty minutes, two or three times a day, to counting fetal movements. After doing this a few times a normal rate can be established which will serve as reference point for subsequent counts. It is suggested that the counting of fetal movements during a subsequent pregnancy be started one month prior to the time in the previous pregnancy when a problem was first detected.

This test has one disadvantage: since every baby goes through a resting period on a regular basis, the counting of movements during one of these periods will not give a clear picture of the baby's condition. In such cases a reduction in fetal movement will not necessarily indicate deteriorating fetal health and unless this is recognized undue anxiety can be created. When reduction in fetal movements is noted the test should be repeated within the next three to four hours, by which time the fetus is likely to have completed its resting period. If the fetal movement count continues to be diminished, you should notify your doctor so a more thorough exam can be undertaken.

As we have seen, there are now a number of tests available that give us considerable clues as to the condition of the fetus. The fetus is no longer isolated from outside observation in the uterine sac but is accessible for evaluation. There is a good understanding of the specificity of these tests. No test is entirely perfect, but when the various tests are utilized together in a way that is appropriate to the individual pregnancy, they can bring reassurance to parents. They can also bring to light developing problems, so that steps can be taken to prevent harm to the baby.

Susan's Story

When our son Alexander was born we knew right away there was a problem — but we didn't know he was going to die. I'd had a C-section in the late afternoon and the hours and night which followed seemed very unreal. After Gene had talked with the doctors at the hospital where Alexander had been taken and had received a diagnosis of our son's condition, he tried to explain it to me. I only wanted to know the bottom line — was our baby going to be okay? With tears in his eyes, he shook his head and answered, "No." Alexander died in Gene's arms that evening.

My physical healing was achieved fairly quickly. But the emotional hurt remained. I knew we wanted to have another baby, but I often found myself vacillating between that desire and the fear of risking another loss. Gene and I had been married 10 years and we had postponed parenthood until things "seemed right." When it took almost a year to conceive, we questioned our decision to wait so long. When Alexander died, we seriously wondered whether or not we'd ever become parents.

Grief turned out to be long and difficult. I was an active participant in the grief process, not wanting to experience it only passively. I was determined to get through the grief process and stay healthy.

One day, well over a year after Alexander's death, I found myself telling a friend that I felt I was luckier than a mutual friend who was unable to get pregnant. I had experienced the joy of being pregnant and giving birth. She hadn't. It surprised me to realize that finally the joy of his too-short existence was greater than the burden of grief.

At last, a year and a half later, I became pregnant again. My emotions ranged from excitement to fear — moment to moment and day to day. Sometimes I could not believe this was finally going to happen. At 15 weeks, I went in for an amniocentesis. A week later I started spotting and an ultrasound revealed that our baby had died.

My grief took a different form this time. I was in absolute shock that this could happen again. I was enraged. Because I had become well acquainted with grief only recently I was not interested in embarking on that path again so soon. I was in the middle of a large project at work and so I used that as a way of escaping from my grief. I became too intensely involved in the project to acknowledge my emotions.

Three weeks later the results of the chromosome study revealed that our baby was a girl — with no chromosome problems. Apparently her death was caused by an infection introduced through amniocentesis. We named her Celeste.

I didn't know what I had wanted to hear — whether Celeste had died because she had a problem similar to Alexander's or whether she had died from some unknown cause. Ultimately I realized that I was powerless to choose what that news would be.

My grief then manifested itself through physical means. I began feeling faint. I would interpret normal feelings in my body as being something drastically wrong. I was sure I had a brain tumor. I was literally filled with fear for my own survival. A physical exam revealed that my symptoms were all in my head — most likely to cover up the pain in my heart from losing Celeste. It was then I realized I couldn't avoid grieving for this baby too.

Because we wanted to be sure everything was okay before we spread the news of this second pregnancy, only our family and very few friends knew of our loss — so acknowledgement of our grief was very limited. I didn't want to risk being seen as a pathetic person and being remembered always with pity.

Losing a child is the most painful thing I have ever experienced. But the pain of a subsequent loss is not twice as bad. It just hurts that much again. Because I was aware of what to expect, it didn't catch me off guard the second time, so I felt more in control.

It took almost a year after our second loss to get pregnant again. And yes, we would choose to have an amniocentesis again, even though the previous one ended in Celeste's death. If we are to accept the good in medical technology then we are bound to also accept the bad. As it turned out, we found out through an ultrasound at nine weeks that I would miscarry — our third loss.

Once more the tears flowed and with the tears a profound sense of the injustice that is present in this world. Somehow I'm still able to have a sense of hope. Maybe it's because I won't take no for an answer. I feel very strongly that Gene and I will one day be parents. This story will not be over until it has a happy ending. We are willing to rewrite the finale to this part of life if we must . . . but not just yet.

Susan Still

Molly's Story

What a difference a day makes. One day my life contained all that I could have wanted. The next day my daughter's short life ended after 36 weeks in my womb. I felt as though my life also had stopped. After the doctor said he couldn't find a heartbeat I was sweating and nauseated. What a horrible feeling — a nightmare come true. Life was a blur for weeks. I felt numb. My anger was so intense and the loss unbelievable. I had never given a thought to the possibility of a stillbirth and I certainly never imagined that it could happen to us.

Soon I found myself pregnant again, quite unexpectedly, only two months after Anna's death. My emotions were so mixed. I longed for my daughter and I wanted this new baby to be her. I was frightened about the pregnancy but I kept telling myself I should be ok because I had already paid my dues. But life offers no guarantees and the nightmare returned.

In the 28th week of my pregnancy my deja vu was complete. Ben died as Anna had died, because of an umbilical accident.

I can still hear the doctor's words of disbelief, "Oh, Molly . . ." My stomach turned. It was totally unbelievable. I felt that I must be an awful person to have had this happen twice. Maybe I wasn't supposed to bear children. Maybe there really was something dreadfully wrong with me.

If I was numb after Anna's death, I was all the more so after Ben died. I don't remember much about that winter. I was very depressed and angry. Fortunately my son and husband were very tolerant of my emotional instability. It was hard for all of us to bear these meaningless deaths.

Both deaths were equally devastating. However I think Ben's death was harder to accept because the disbelief was more profound. My feelings of failure intensified and my sense of hope diminished. My self-esteem was shot.

We still wanted another child because of our wonderful experience with our older child Sam. Also, I felt a need to prove to someone — I don't know who — that I could pull this off and bring a live baby to term. After all, having a baby is supposed to be no big deal. Any woman can have a child.

I became pregnant again 10 months after Ben's death only to miscarry for the third time, at 8 weeks. I didn't need to be kicked in the face again, but I didn't feel like I had any choice but to try again. So we kept trying, all the time wondering how we could be so stupid as to risk being so terribly disappointed again.

But desperation can make one persistent. I became pregnant once more and once again was petrified with fear about what was to come. I couldn't feel happy or excited. I didn't know what to do, since I felt like I had tried everything in my two previous pregnancies to no avail. I became quite superstitious. Still I never gave up hope that, as long as I remained pregnant, there was hope that my baby would be born alive.

At 36 weeks, Margaret was born — alive and perfect. I was happy and sad and all mixed up. But a miracle had happened for us and I remain grateful.

I am sure people thought we were crazy to keep trying to enlarge our family. But how could we explain our needs and wants to them when they had no way of knowing what we'd been through? I guess we just needed to find the hope that we knew must be there for us. We were so low, we needed some way to get up out of the hole we were in.

Certain family members and friends were wonderfully supportive. Others just were not supportive at all and that added to the hurt. Stillbirth is such a difficult loss to explain, and it is hard for others to realize what a real and painful experience it is for parents. I desperately wanted Anna and Ben to be recognized as real children who had actually lived. It was, and still is, hard to help certain individuals to acknowledge that.

Three years have passed since the nightmare began. Time has been the greatest healer. My Compassionate Friends group has been my greatest help and support. The birth of Margaret has improved my self-esteem and mood greatly. But at the same time her birth has tended to intensify my sense of loss, for it has made me realize all the more keenly the absence of Anna and Ben. Rob has been wonderfully helpful in reminding me that we can't have what we have lost, but that because of our loss, we will love the children we have all the more.

I encourage all who find themselves in the same situation not to lose hope. Fortunately time passes and the sun does shine again.

Molly Olson

Chapter 4
Living Through Another Pregnancy

THIS DAY

something began for me that day
something ended for me that day
that day everyone was silent
soft sunlight shone on maple leaves
angels were yawning that day
a day like today
a day like yesterday
nothing began for anyone else that day
nothing ended for anyone else that day
alone I crossed a railroad crossing
and crossed back over again
and crossed again
I then crouched in the middle of the tracks
and looked down the tracks at the setting sun

that was a day like today
a day like tomorrow
I kept quiet, unable to weep this day
somebody moves around in the womb
something begins for me this day
something ends for me this day
pods of peas are snapped
a kitten falls into the river this day
a day of death amid life

by Shuntaro Tanikawa

Finding Out You're Pregnant

"I felt like a kid trying to do the impossible."

"I couldn't wait to get pregnant. That's all I could think about. For the first three days after I found out I was pregnant I was elated. After that I was scared to death. I wanted an abortion."

"I didn't want to tell anybody that I was pregnant so they wouldn't know I failed again. That way if I aborted I would be the only one to know."

"I wanted an abortion because I could tell I couldn't handle the emotions I was going through. My doctor wanted to give me some medication for a cold, but I refused to take the medication for fear it would hurt the baby. On the one hand I wanted to kill the baby; on the other hand I didn't want the baby to get hurt."

"I decided not to tell my family and friends because I didn't want them to worry about me, or to be disappointed if something went wrong."

"I was afraid to tell people I was pregnant because I didn't want them to think I was just trying to replace the baby that died."

"I was elated to find out I was pregnant. I just walked around grinning. I couldn't understand why women who had experienced a loss were so scared — until I reached the point in my pregnancy when I was supposed to be able to feel the baby move. From that point on I was a nervous wreck."

"I didn't want to admit to myself or anyone else that I could be pregnant. I put off calling the doctor's office for an appointment until I was almost five months pregnant. When the nurse said the earliest available appointment was four weeks away, I panicked! I needed to see the doctor today!"

Taking Care of Yourself

"I did absolutely everything right during my last pregnancy. I was a model patient. I ate right, took my vitamins, didn't drink . . . not even a little. And still my baby died. This time I'm more casual. Being perfect didn't pay off."

"Even though I was careful last time, and nothing I did caused my baby to die — at least as far as my doctor could tell — I'm not taking any chances this time. People think I'm a fanatic. But if this baby dies, I don't want it to be my fault."

The two statements above are opposites. The first one recognizes that there are no guarantees, and takes a "what's the use" attitude. The other says, "If I do everything right I won't be held accountable for anything that may go wrong." To some degree both statements make sense. But in both statements there is something missing.

As a parent, no matter how thoroughly you rationalize your action you will continue to feel guilty if something happens to your baby. There is no getting around it. What both of these women are trying to do, as indicated by their statements, is to protect themselves from pain . . . just in case. It won't work.

Because you are a responsible caring person your job as the mother of your unborn child is to provide for, to nurture, and to protect this child so it can receive the best possible start. That does not mean you have to be paranoid about everything you do, but it does mean you will care enough not to take unnecessary risks that could put your baby's future in jeopardy. This is what all mothers should be willing to do, not just mothers who have had a baby die.

For some mothers pregnancy will be easy. For others it will require a continual conscious commitment to another life. For example, if you are a nonsmoker, not smoking because it could possibly harm your unborn baby will present no challenge to you. But if you are a smoker, deciding not to smoke for your baby's sake is a burden that may be difficult. Or, some women will have to stay in bed for most of their pregnancy because of complications while others will be able to enjoy an active pregnancy.

Along with wanting to do the best you can is knowing what is best for you and your baby and how to make this pregnancy a safe journey for your little passenger.

When we mention the word safe, you might find yourself getting tense. Your jaw gets tight and the knot in your stomach returns. How can anyone guarantee you that if you do all the right things that your baby will be safe? Your past experience has been your educator on absolutes. Nobody can fool you again.

The word safe is relative. On one hand you dare your caregiver to give you absolutes, on the other hand you may be desperate for assurance. Obstetrics at best is an art, not a science. We, too, are frustrated by not being able to make perfect predictions.

Our lives are filled with opposites; there's yes and no, black and white, day and night, birth and death, and joy and sorrow. Our words probably sound very wishy washy. Our sentences are filled with usually, probably in most cases, almost always. The only always that we can guarantee is the baby will be delivered.

Every day we learn more. Every day a new theory takes the place of an old one. Every day we come closer to fully understanding the biological relationship between mother and child. This is probably difficult for you to accept. You want assurances. Clear, concrete promises that if you do everything right you won't have to go through another loss.

We offer you the following information to help you do the best job you can. The information is backed by current research. Based on that knowledge we assure you these suggestions will at least reduce the risks, or increase your chances of having a healthy baby. But remember, your caregiver is the best person to give you individual medical advice to assure a healthy outcome for both you and your baby.

***"But I know someone who smokes and her baby was nine pounds."* That's right. And some people walk across the street on a red light and don't get hit by a car.**

1. An ideal weight gain during pregnancy is 25-35 pounds. This is not time to go on a starvation diet. The only way your baby eats is through your mouth. Your baby cannot live off your excess fat. If you are a vegetarian check with a nutritionist to make sure you are getting all the nutrients your body requires to nourish your unborn child.

2. Avoid saunas and long hot tub baths. This can increase your internal body temperature which can lead to problems in your baby's development.

3. Exercise is good for you during pregnancy, but should be done in moderation. Exercise can not only increase your body temperature and therefore cause development problems in your baby but also temporarily reduce the oxygen supply to your baby. Mothers who are in fairly rigorous athletic training tend to have smaller babies. It has been suggested that you do 2/3 the amount of exercise you generally did before pregnancy.

4. Don't smoke. Smoking constricts blood vessels, including the ones that carry oxygenated blood to the uterus causing decreased oxygen supply to the baby. Babies born to mothers who smoke will be of lower birth weight than those who don't smoke. The more you smoke the greater the hazard to your baby.

5. If you eat raw meat or handle feces while cleaning your cat's litter box you can expose your baby to a condition called Toxoplasmosis. Though the majority of women who have tested out to have Toxoplasmosis during pregnancy have healthy babies, the affected children may exhibit degrees of blindness, mental retardation, jaundice or anemia.

6. Megadoses of vitamins can cause deformities in your baby. Eating a well balanced diet and supplementing with prenatal vitamins should be able to cover all the needed vitamins your body and baby need during pregnancy and lactation. If you have a vitamin deficiency your caregiver can advise you on taking additional vitamins. Too much of a good thing can be harmful.

7. Try to avoid eating foods that contain additives. Though the studies that link additives to deformities in babies have all been done on animals, consider it a safety precaution for your baby.

8. Don't take *any* medications (including over-the-counter drugs) without first consulting your caregiver. Even if you have taken medications during a previous pregnancy or someone you knew had, don't take a chance. The list of potentially harmful drugs if taken during pregnancy continues to rise. What we thought was safe in the past may no longer be considered safe. For example, diuretics that were commonly prescribed for women for water retention are now found to cause low birth weight infants, possible limb deformities, jaundice or hypoglycemia.

It is important to remember that there are two people involved when taking medications during pregnancy. Sometimes the benefits of taking the medication for the mother outweigh the possible risk to the baby.

Questions that need to be considered before taking medications are:

a. Do you really need the medication, or is there something else you could do to alleviate the need for it, i.e. change your diet, get more exercise, quit work, etc.

b. Is there some other medication that could be prescribed that would be less hazardous to the baby?

c. Do the benefits of taking the medication for the mother outweigh the possible risks to the baby?

9. Drinking alcohol during pregnancy can cause your baby to be born with a defect called Fetal Alcohol Syndrome. Babies born with this condition exhibit defects such as mental retardation, facial malformation, low birth weight and heart defects. Because of the brain development that happens early in pregnancy the most hazardous time for drinking may be the very early part of the pregnancy. There is not conclusive evidence on the precise dose of alcohol that endangers the baby, though it is known that "heavy" drinkers place their baby's health in extreme jeopardy. To be safe abstinence may be your best choice.

10. Emotional stress may play a role in harming your unborn child. Studies have shown that women who demonstrated high levels of anxiety had increased incidence of: miscarriage, preeclampsia, fetal distress, complications at birth and low birth weight babies. The most important factor that can alleviate stress related problems is addressing the underlying causes for the anxiety before or during pregnancy.

Above all, do no harm.
Hippocratic Oath

Feelings During Pregnancy

"I decided it would be bad luck to think positively about this pregnancy. I'm a born loser."

"I know I'm making myself as miserable as possible. That way I know everything will be okay. If I suffer enough now I won't have to suffer later."

"My husband told me to stop imagining the worst, for fear I would cause the worst to happen. I know he will blame me if something goes wrong this time."

"I can't stand to be around pregnant women who haven't had a baby die. They are so naive. If they only knew . . ."

"One of the women at work told me she wasn't going to give me a baby gift this time. She said I already got one from her last time."

"Everyone seems truly relieved that I'm pregnant. Now they think they don't have to talk about my dead baby anymore. It's like they're saying 'Whew, I'm glad that's over.' "

"I'm afraid to appear too happy. If I seem happy people will think I'm no longer sad and that I have forgotten my dead baby. I will never forget."

"I went around the house getting everything in order just in case I died. I made sure all my important papers were easy for my husband to find."

"I don't want to hold another baby unless it's mine. I can't stand seeing new moms with their babies. It's so unfair. I've been trying to have a live baby for three years and those mothers were successful after only ten months."

"If this baby dies, I want to die too."

"We loved my body while I was pregnant the first time. This time I feel like my body is just a vessel."

"I don't think too much about this pregnancy. It's not that I don't care, because I do. I'm just not excited like I was the last time."

"After the results of the amniocentesis came back and everything looked fine, I then worried that my baby's death would be from a cord accident."

What is meant to be a special time in a woman's life may take on quite a different reality for you once you have suffered the loss of a child. You may look back to the former pregnancy and remember how thrilled you were with every new change in your body. Pregnancy was a wonderful time filled with idealistic dreams of the larger family you were soon to become. But all that is past now. No more do you approach each new stage of pregnancy with a sense of wonder and excitement. Instead of reveling in the joy of an unfolding miracle, you may find yourself treading cautiously and fearfully — one step at a time — feeling nothing but relief as each step brings you closer to the end.

The comments on the preceding page, shared by women during their subsequent pregnancies, reveal ambivalent feelings which you too may encounter from time to time. When these women were asked if they had any regrets about their subsequent pregnancy, they all expressed the wish that they had been able to enjoy the pregnancy more. They were sorry that they hadn't retained positive memories similar to those they held close from the period during the previous pregnancy before they learned that their little child had died.

None of us knows ahead of time how long we will have a child with us. It may be only for the span of time that the child is growing inside. It may be for only four days after the birth, or four years. We just don't know. But if we can learn to appreciate what we *do* have while we have it, at least we won't have to regret that we can think of nothing positive to remember about this little person's life-before-birth. This baby you are now carrying also deserves to be remembered warmly for the joy that he brings you while still inside you. And because the tragic conclusion of your past pregnancy will tend to cloud your experience with this and future pregnancies, you will need consciously to make happen what came more naturally before.

Of course you won't be able to make this experience exactly like the earlier one. But if you are willing to give up the notion that nothing can replace the experience you had, you will find that in this subsequent pregnancy life can unfold in ways that are new and different — and every bit as positive.

Times that may be particularly hard during this next pregnancy

1. The first trimester, especially if you have had miscarriages in the past. Most women breathe a sigh of relief when they know at least they won't miscarry.

2. The first time you hear the baby's heartbeat. What a relief, but you may be filled with memories of hearing your dead baby's heartbeat.

3. Having an amniocentesis or any other test that may cause problems . . . and then waiting for the results to come back.

4. Waking up before the baby does and not feeling her move. These poor babies should not have to perform all the time. They, too, need sleep.

Note: Some subsequent pregnancy groups have dopplers to loan if you are overly anxious about the baby not moving so you can tune in to the baby's heartbeat if you aren't feeling her move. You can also go to your doctor's office or the maternity unit of your hospital just to have fetal heart tones checked or have a non-stress test run if you are really concerned.

5. The time during your pregnancy when there was a hint of a problem with your baby's health.

6. The anniversary date of your baby's birth and death.

7. Holidays, just because it reminds you that you weren't suppose to be pregnant on this holiday, but a mother holding a baby.

To bring anything into your life,
imagine that it is already there

Sex During Pregnancy

If you have recently suffered the loss of your child you may have found your sex life diminished by the pangs of grief. You may be avoiding sex altogether because the mere thought of seeking or experiencing pleasure when you are absorbed by your grief is unacceptable to you. You may find yourself thinking, 'How can I allow myself to have fun when my child lies dead?' Many parents share this feeling. Or, even if you have been engaging in sexual intercourse — in a frantic attempt to conceive again — you are probably not able to enter freely into the enjoyment of making love.

Once the desired pregnancy is achieved other problems may arise to make sex a continued stressful experience rather than an enjoyable release for you.

Some of the sex related problems of grieving parents are typical of pregnancy in general. Though some couples enjoy sex during pregnancy as much as they do when they are not pregnant, and maybe even more, others for various reasons find sex less pleasurable. We had assumed that parents who had experienced the death of their child at birth would tend to avoid sexual intercourse during a subsequent pregnancy for fear of possible harm to their unborn baby, even though there is no evidence to support this fear. Our assumption was based on statements bereaved parents have made about not wanting to be responsible for risking the death of another child. We were wrong, however. We found that most bereaved parents do have intercourse, though not as often, and admit that the experience is not as pleasurable as it was during the previous pregnancy. It seems that the same irrational fears that haunt the subsequent pregnancy in general also take their toll on lovemaking.

Because you may be concerned unnecessarily about the affect of sex during pregnancy, based on information offered in the past, we have included the updated information below. We hope this information will help you to feel more comfortable about making love if that is your desire.

1. If you are in good health, there is little danger that sexual intercourse will lead to infection that could harm your baby. If you are concerned about this possibility, use of a condom is recommended.

2. Having an orgasm is okay and is not likely to cause premature labor unless you have had a history of premature labor. Most women experience some mild contractions following an orgasm. That is okay.

3. Nipple stimulation should also be avoided if premature labor is a concern.

4. If you or your doctor is concerned that the prostaglandin hormones present in the semen might cause premature labor, a condom can be worn.

5. The only sex act that is strictly advised against is forcefully blowing air into the vagina. This is a concern in any pregnancy. Blowing air into the vagina can cause an air embolus, which could be fatal to the woman.

6. There is not reason to abstain from intercourse unless you have been advised to do so for medical reasons, or unless

you choose to. If abstinence is advised it may be for one or more of the following reasons:

a. a history of miscarriage.
b. undiagnosed vaginal bleeding or known placenta previa. (The placenta is lying across the opening of the cervix.)
c. chronic infection of the reproductive system. (This applies to your partner as well.)

If your physician advises against sexual intercourse during your pregnancy find out exactly what the doctor means. Are you not to have penetration during intercourse or is orgasm the concern? This information will help you decide if masturbation would be a safe alternative. If the topic of sex is not brought up by your doctor, you should initiate it. It is important for you to know the facts so that you don't base your decisions on unfounded assumptions.

Loving, touching, kissing, fondling, or just being close are all part of lovemaking. For some couples these forms of intimacy will be all that is needed during pregnancy. Just feeling loved and cared for will be sufficient. But you can't assume that your partner is feeling the same way you are. It's possible he also has some unspoken fears, or unmet needs. The most helpful advice we can give you here is to talk with each other about your individual needs. Open communication is essential. This may be a perfect time for more creative lovemaking between you and your partner.

**When you cannot find peace in yourself
it is useless to look for it elsewhere.**

La Rochefoucauld

"Mommy, do we get to take this baby home?"

"Gee, dad . . . a brother, that's great, but is he alive?"

"We have a new sister at our house. She hasn't died yet."

"Is it okay with Anna (the dead sibling) if Christie plays with her toys?"

"I wish Elizabeth was alive, I'm sure she would have been nicer to me than Carrie is."

How Children Respond to Another Pregnancy

Children in the family are also touched by a younger sibling's death. They won't grieve in quite the same way as their parents but indeed they will grieve. In general we find that, in their grief, young children tend to reflect the level of emotional development of the adults in their family. If the parents are open and able to communicate their feelings the children will be open and communicative also.

As you read the following comments remember that each child is just as unique in his or her grief as is any individual adult. One child will be affected in a certain way while another will show different reactions to the sibling's death.

When you become pregnant again you may discover that your young child now thinks you will soon be happy again. Because they have never experienced a profound loss of a relationship yet, and their emotional development has not matured they are incapable of understanding that getting a new baby is not like getting a new puppy after one dies. The child does see this new baby as a replacement and may feel much relieved, believing — or hoping — that this new pregnancy will end your sorrow.

These children have had a different life experience than their peers though and will reflect that in their matter-of-fact way of acknowledging that there are three kinds of babies to have — girl babies, boy babies and dead babies. Don't be surprised if you hear them ask questions such as, "Will this one be born dead too?" or, "Will we get to take this one home?"

The child may not be pleased at all to learn that you are pregnant again, because of the fear of either losing you to your grief, if this new baby should die (a repeat of the child's recent experience), or losing you to the new baby, if the baby should survive. The child may feel like he or she is in a no-win situation.

81

Some children have reacted to the death of a sibling by becoming overly anxious about the mother's health during the subsequent pregnancy. If for some reason you need to be hospitalized during the pregnancy make every attempt to talk with your child on the phone or have the child come to the hospital for visits to reassure the child that you will be returning.

After the baby is born your older child may show some change from normal behavior. Some parents have reported that their school-age child's school work was affected for a while. Others have noticed their children started doing negative things to draw attention to themselves. These reactions are not uncommon for any sibling, whether they've experienced a sibling death before or not.

Many children have also mirrored the same anxieties that parents show about the survival of this new baby by constantly checking on the sleeping infant. For the most part however, siblings seem to see these new little people as "special," just like you will. The older children will adjust readily if they are given plenty of love and attention without having to demand it. If the children are school age, make sure you keep in close contact with their teachers and counselors.

Mommy, where do helium balloons go?
Up, up and away.
Do they go up to heaven?
Yes, I think so.
Then, this can go to baby Holly.
    Erik Stanbro

Support Groups

We weep together
We laugh together
We hope together

It is said that at least 50% of one's personal stress can be relieved by talking things through with another person. Most of us can only go so far trying to think through a problem alone. Even after we have worked through a problem on our own, and have actually done a reasonable job considering the limitations of a monologue, we have the potential for even deeper insight if we allow other people to ask questions and to make suggestions which challenge us to go further in our thinking.

So, it's quite normal to need other people to see you through another tough time. Any friend who is willing to listen will be of some help, but a person who has "been there" herself will be even better. A self-help subsequent pregnancy group may be just what you need right now.

Some doctors are reluctant to refer their patients to a support group because they are concerned that the client's fears will be increased rather than decreased when they hear about complications that other women have experienced during their pregnancies. It is true that you will learn about other possible problems that you otherwise might not have known about. That can't be helped. But the advantages of a self-help support group for couples during a subsequent pregnancy far outweigh the disadvantages.

No pregnancy should be a lonely experience. But if you have chosen not to talk with other pregnant women because you're feeling gloom and doom, and you can't relate to their naive and carefree attitudes about pregnancy, you may have sentenced yourself to a pregnancy locked into an emotional solitary confinement. In a support group, on the other hand, you will meet parents who will understand and validate your fears, but who at the same time will also help you talk about the positive aspects of your pregnancy. You will learn how others have handled unpleasant pregnancy-related experiences such as dealing with insensitive people. Some women have been grateful that in a support group their husbands were able to meet other pregnant women who were just as "crazy" during pregnancy as they themselves were. Or if you are harboring a secret fear that something is really wrong with your baby, and you have been afraid to consult the doctor about your concern, you can bet that someone in the group will give you the encouragement you need to call your doctor. She may even be willing to go with you to talk to the doctor if you need a companion.

The support doesn't end when the baby is born. It continues throughout the early parenting months when bonding and grief are still major concerns. And you will probably have gained new and lasting friendships as a result of your support group experience.

A list of some of the nationally known programs which sponsor local groups is found on page 117. Your hospital social service department, local childbirth education groups or mental health association will be able to put you in touch with specific groups in your local area. If there is no support group in your area, you might consider starting one. There are probably other couples in your own neighborhood who need you as much as you need them.

Laughter

**Those who do not know how to weep
with their whole heart
Don't know how to laugh either**

Golda Meir

Laughter is like singing. It can fill a room with sweet smiles. When you laugh watch how the laughter infects those around you. It's hard not to join right in. There is nothing so freeing and filling as a rolling belly laugh, when you think your sides are going to burst if you continue and your ribs ache when you are through. It's not just a "hee, hee, hee" but a "ho, ho, ho." And what wonderful medicine laughter can be to the aching heart and ailing body. Norman Cousins writes in *Anatomy of an Illness* how he laughed himself back to health when doctors had given up all hope of curing him of a catastrophic illness. Albert Schweitzer also knew how to use laughter as an antidote for the stresses of work which he and his young fellow doctors and nurses encountered at the Schweitzer Hospital. He administered daily doses of humor during their evening meal together. They would all return to work rejuvenated and cleansed by laughter.

Most likely there was a time after your baby died when you thought you would never be able to laugh again, when nothing seemed very funny and seeing others having a good time only made you more withdrawn. Laughter is extremely important and therapeutic in times like these. Laughter needs to find a place in your life again. If your life is lacking in laughter don't wait for your new baby to make you laugh again. There are things you can do right away that will help you to recover a vital sense of humor.

The merry heart works like a doctor
Proverbs 17:22

Some of the most memorable and special evenings in our subsequent pregnancy support groups have been those during which parents dared to tell about absurd things that happened to them during their initial grief. Or they would describe their own bizarre behavior during their "unconscious" days, like putting the phone in the refrigerator!

These are experiences bereaved parents will probably never share with "outsiders" because they suspect an outsider would think that they were crazy. But let one parent start a conversation about "my most embarrassing moment" and soon the whole group will be rolling on the floor, one-upping each other with forgiving stories. Forgiving? Yes. Earlier in the grief process such incidents were painful reminders to the bereaved how much their own lives were out of control or how terribly bewildered they felt by what seemed to be the whole world's lack of understanding of grief. Now that they have reached the point of permitting themselves to laugh, their anger has begun to mellow, and they are able to forgive themselves and others.

There is no limit to the variety of absurd behavior of which you are capable in your grief. For example, you may find you've become superstitious for the first time in your life. You may have an irrational compulsion to drive a different route to the doctor's office, avoiding the route you used during your last pregnancy. Or you may imagine that your unborn baby will hear you arguing with your spouse and decide to die rather than be born into this bickering family. Such responses are completely irrational . . . but very real to you if you're the one experiencing them. Make light of them. Temporary insanity is acceptable.

In the early days of your grief you had no control over your feelings or reactions to events, but now you do. You can choose what you want to make of a situation. You can allow yourself to be devastated, depressed, or angered or you can choose to lighten up and laugh at the absurdity of it all.

Labor's moving fast . . . we knew it would. It did the last time. And because I knew it was unlikely that the hospital would have a gown big enough to fit my oversized body so I could join Deb in the delivery room, I told the staff early of last year's problems . . . One nurse wheeled Deb into the delivery room. The other nurse handed me a scrub suit to put on. It wouldn't fit. So she handed me two patient gowns and told me to go put them on. I did . . . quickly. When I returned she said, "Not good enough. You have to take off your clothes first and then put the gowns on." At this point I knew that my only objective was to be beside Deb when our baby was born. They could have handed me a stork outfit and I would have obliged them. I did what the nurse said. I sandwiched myself in between two patient gowns, front and back, I donned my hat, shoe covers and mask and headed for the delivery room. As I entered the delivery room our doctor wheeled around in his stool to greet me and when he saw my outfit he said, "Well, if it isn't 'Friar Tuck,'" He then broke into a roar of laughter.

★ ★ ★ ★

My pregnancy was nine months of concern for my baby and increasing discomfort for me. The last few months were spent in bed due to the pain from my abdominal cerclage. My doctor had been a gift from heaven. She was so understanding and patient through some very trying times with me. I wanted to work, but couldn't work. I was uncomfortable, but I didn't want to take any medication that would harm my baby. I wanted to remain in bed, but I couldn't stand being still. At last we were finally near the end of what seemed like the longest pregnancy on record even though we were actually a few weeks ahead of schedule

I wanted to do something to show my doctor that I still had a sense of humor after all those months. It was to be my sign to her that down deep I knew everything would be all right. I decided that I would find some stickers with humorous sayings on them and fasten them to my belly alongside my old C-section scar where my doctor would discover them just before the surgery. I sent friends to search for the stickers with the most appropriate messages.

As Russ and I waited together before the surgery which would bring Matthew into the world, we were both giddy with delight that we had thought of this great joke to play on our doctor. We tried to imagine what she would do and we wondered if the nurses would be upset at this breach of hospital decorum.

87

The joke couldn't have worked better. The timing was perfect — and so was the outcome of our pregnancy.

Men

By observing how men grieve following the death of their babies we are reminded of the strong influence of socially assigned roles in the lives of all of us. If you remember that our society assigns to men the traditional family roles of problem solver, provider, protector, competitor, and leader it then becomes easier to understand why men often "appear" to their wives and to others to be less emotional in their expression of grief. And it is easy to understand why these same actions and outward expressions by men carry over into a subsequent pregnancy as well.

In most cases a man will tend not to express the same degree of fear for the safety of the new baby as does his wife. This could be because he did not have as close a relationship with the baby that died as did the wife, thus making it difficult for him to mirror her strong feelings. A more likely explanation is that he is performing the role he believes he is supposed to play in their relationship. How can he be strong, supportive and protective if he talks of doom, gloom and vulnerability? He considers such behaviors to be inconsistent with his perceived role. However, after the birth many men do admit to a sense of relief that suggests the presence of hidden or unacknowledged anxiety during the pregnancy.

If you are the father-to-be, you know how difficult it can be to try to carry on a conversation with a spouse who keeps worrying that the new baby is doomed to die. How do you respond when she says, "Our baby is not going to make it; I just have this feeling about it." Do you say, "Gee I'm sorry to hear that," or would you ignore her statement and say, "Would you turn the T.V. to another channel, please?" All kidding aside, these responses express your frustration in dealing with a partner who is so pessimistic about an outcome which you both desperately want.

She doesn't want to feel that way either. And if she could climb out of her pit of doubt and despair right now she would. We suggest that you just hold her tenderly during these times, allow her to express herself without feeling she will be put down for her outbursts, and if she is talking about some reasonably valid concerns help her follow up on them. Go to the doctor with her. Be as supportive as you can be. Remind yourself that there will also be good days to share.

Make sure you get your needs met too. Talk with other men who are also going through a subsequent pregnancy. You will see that what you are dealing with is quite normal. And don't be afraid to tell your wife about your own fears. She needs to know what you are feeling too. Give her a chance to be supportive of you.

My dearest wife and friend,

How can I tell you the joy and gratitude I feel tonight after seeing our third son born? He's truly God's masterpiece made through us.

After Benjamin died, I thought it was unfair that I should even ask you to try to get pregnant again because of the chance that we might have to experience such pain once more. We knew our chances were one in four that our tragedy could be repeated. I'd never considered myself a gambler.

I remember the many hours of weeping and sorting through the emotions of letting Benjamin go. He was our first born. His birth brought me a new role to play. I thought I would be his teacher, but he was so much wiser. In his few months with us, he taught me how precious life is. He taught me to be grateful for what we have now and not to wait for something else to make me happy.

When he died I felt for a long time that my life had ceased to have meaning. Even through all of your pain you were able to still care for me. Thank you for sticking it out with me.

But we continued to want a child to love and to grow with. And because we knew the chances of our not encountering the same genetic disorder were better if we didn't make a baby together, we opted for artificial insemination. I knew that you wanted to be pregnant again and artificial insemination seemed the logical way to go.

I can still hear you ranting and raving at the thought that someone else was controlling our lovemaking. You couldn't work when you were ovulating and every period was like another death. Though I didn't have any problems with the concept of AID, it just seemed so cold and impersonal — a complete contradiction to how we would have made a baby together. After 6 months of that disruption in our lives we decided to discontinue the artificial insemination and consider another alternative.

We chose adoption, but not without ambivalent feelings. Adoption, we had heard, could take forever. Besides that it seemed to us, at first, to imply failure. Remember how angry we were about having to prove to others that we would be fit parents? This whole ordeal seemed to be such an insult. Look at all we would have to go through after all we had been through.

Thank God for your sense of humor and willingness to put up with all that.

But our miracle finally happened. With a knock on the door a new baby entered our lives. Michael, just two days old, came in to fill our healing hearts 13 months after Benjamin's death. He came to teach me the art of being responsible. He gently taught me to care again and to know that perfect is an "imperfect" word.

It was Michael that gaves us the courage to try to become pregnant again ourselves. He represented some security for us. At least we knew we had one child at home if we were to have another baby die. And we figured that nothing that might happen to us could be any worse than what we'd already experienced. Meeting another couple with a background similar to ours and a subsequent success story gave us hope. Maybe it would help to look at the odds in a positive way — saying that we had a 75% chance to succeed rather than a 25% chance of getting burned again. I suspect that it was our happiness because of the joy that Michael had brought us that made us crazy enough to decide to try again when he was barely four months old.

We decided that we would try for no longer than one year. Two months later — bingo! Our joy was beyond belief. We couldn't understand the fears that others had in a subsequent pregnancy. We prided ourselves on our positive attitude. We weren't the least bit concerned, were we?

Then came the 20th week, when we should expect to feel the baby's first movements. Because Benjamin's problem had been a muscle disorder, we needed this new baby to reassure us with good strong kicks. He hardly moved at all. This baby felt no different than Benjamin. The days seemed endless as we counted fetal movements that never quite matched up to the doctor's expectations. The amount of ice cream we consumed to get our baby to move cost me 20 pounds. (It was all worth it, by the way.)

Some days your doom and gloom would get to me. It was all I could do to keep optimistic myself without your talking about the possibility that the baby might die. You'd just hope that this baby would not have to live as long as Benjamin, or you'd wonder how much more you needed to suffer before you had paid your price. It seemed that you were wanting to get the death over with, since you were almost sure that it was going to happen anyway. I felt my job was to keep your spirits up and be the optimistic one.

I'd go to work and listen to my office-mate talking about his pregnant wife and how much his baby was moving. And I would quietly fret knowing that ours just wasn't matching up. Oh, I'd try to be cheerful and make light conversation, but my desire was to get the hell out of there. I remember I didn't talk about this pregnancy like I did when you were pregnant with Benjamin. Because our friends thought we were crazy to try again, it was hard to talk to them about how scared we felt at times. I was sure they would just say we asked for it.

I was irritated by your flippant attitude about this baby. No, you didn't want to get the bassinet out, and the nursery preparations took all of one hour. I wondered how I was going to deal with you if you went a couple of weeks over your due date. You were like a time bomb just waiting to explode. It was so different from how you felt about Benjamin's pregnancy. Were you just too afraid to hope? It seemed to me that if we just thought positive thoughts everything would be all right. Pretty male of me, huh? I was sure I could be happy if only you would be optimistic.

The day finally arrived. Our child was to be born. You were as cool as a cucumber. You knew everything was going to be all right. For you, all those fears of doom and gloom seemed to melt away. I was the one who now needed the reassurance. I was anything but calm. This was the moment of truth that I didn't want to have to face. Could I deal with whatever was presented to us?

You were wheeled into the delivery room to be prepared for a cesarean birth. Pat and I donned our scrub outfits. I promptly sat on my glasses and one lens popped out. Maggie, I'm blind without my glasses. I wasn't going to be able to see our child born. Pat searched for some tape to hold me together through the birth. I could imagine the lens popping out just as our baby was born. My panic was barely under control.

When we joined you in the delivery room I remember you looking up at me and laughing at my makeshift spectacles. You immediately saw through my brave exterior and lovingly kidded me.

Within minutes after surgery had begun, the doctor held up a screaming, wriggling son for us to see. You squealed

91

and cried for joy. I wanted to believe, but was afraid. I had what you might call a good case of guarded optimism. Whenever anyone came close I introduced our son, and then asked, "Well, what do you think? Do you think he's all right?"

Yes, Maggie, I'm sure he's all right. And I'm sure we'll be all right too. Benjamin's pregnancy and birth had been fresh like a summer day. We had no concept of pain then. Joseph's pregnancy and birth was more special. Because we didn't close our eyes to what we had learned from our past we were able to share at a depth we have never plumbed before.

Whatever the future holds for us we know we will be all right. We know we can handle whatever we must.

> I love you,
> Gary

And Joseph, I say smiling,
Teaches me joy without much trying,
He just lies there with a grin,
And for some reason I join right in.

Are you sure he's all right?

Healthy, pink, screaming . . . that's my boy.
But, are you sure he's all right?
Looks good, don't you think?
I'm 95% convinced.
What do you think?
He's fine. You'll see.
But are you sure? How can you tell?
Just look at him!
I know, but I just want to be sure.
Are you sure he's all right?
That's my boy!

Is the Sex of Your Next Baby Important?

"We already have two boys. I wanted a girl, but it turned out to be another boy. When he died, I immediately wanted to have another baby and it had to be a boy."

"I didn't care what it was as long as it was healthy. No, it didn't even have to be healthy. Just alive."

"I've got three girls. Friends say, 'Oh good, you'll finally get your boy. How nice.' I don't think it's nice at all. I'm scared to death. You see, both of my babies that died were boys."

"Everyone wants this baby to be a girl to replace the one that died. We already have a boy. Another boy would be just fine with me. I don't want another girl to take my daughter's place. I don't want another daughter to wear her clothes. She was so special — such a charmer. I've had my girl."

"I'm afraid to have a boy. What if he looks just like the boy that died? I'm afraid I'll get confused."

"It's important that we have a girl. The chances of a girl dying from the same problem are much less."

"I want this baby to be a boy and I want him to look exactly like the one that died. He was beautiful. He looked just like my husband."

"I want to have twins. A boy to replace the one that died, and a girl so we don't have to go through this again."

Parents of dead babies are no less likely than parents of live babies to have a specific preference for the sex of their next child. But the reasons for preferring either a boy or a girl may seem even more compelling for those who have had a child die.

The reasons for your own personal preference may not be obvious even to well-meaning friends and relatives, and these persons may make completely unfounded assumptions about your preference. For example, if your surviving child is a boy, they may assume that you will certainly want a girl this time. Or if the boy who died was your only child, they may assume that you still want to have a boy the next time — to replace the child that died. Your friends' chances of being right in their assumptions are no better than 50/50.

It is easy to understand why a woman's fears might be greater if, having given birth to two live girls and two dead boys, she now finds herself pregnant with another boy. Though her friends will be ready to rejoice upon hearing the news that she is carrying a baby boy, the prospect may be anything but comforting to her. They are thinking of the future while she is still dealing with the past. Amnesia would be a welcomed panacea for this woman.

You may find yourself wishing for a boy rather than a girl or vice versa because you imagine the one sex or the other will make it easier to tolerate this pregnancy. It sounds reasonable. If you think your chances are better for a good outcome if you are carrying a girl rather than a boy you will most likely express that preference. Logic in this case is not based on scientific facts, but who said it has to be?

Usually, toward the end of the pregnancy the sex of the child seems less important. By then you mostly just want a baby.

The use of ultrasound or amniocentesis to determine the sex of the baby even before birth has helped many parents to deal with disappointment and fear and to simply get used to the sex of their child apart from the trauma of the birth itself. Confirmation of the baby's sex has also helped some to start relating to their unborn baby more as an individual.

An important thing to know is that even though parents start our preferring a specific sex, they usually wind up well pleased with the outcome, whatever it is. The complete acceptance of this child is not always immediate, but it does come.

You were six days old.
Inside I carry another child
as once I carried you.
When I feel the kicks and moves
I remember feeling you.
The fear tears at me inside.
Could it happen again
as it happened to you?
I ache as the time gets closer
to the time that you were born.
Will this one be eight weeks
early too? Will I lose this
child as I lost you?

Barbara Melling

94

ONE SUNDAY AFTERNOON

One Sunday afternoon
You saw my tears
  Precipitous and sobbing from my eyes,
Too fierce to be ashamed,
Too wounded to be stealthy,
Too sudden to be announced,
And while the water washed your hands and face
  You held me close
To siphon out the pain.

One Sunday afternoon
You saw my tears
  And like an anxious mother asked:
"What brings such weeping?"
  And even as you asked for reasons
The torrents disappeared.
  Only stains of tears remained.

What do reasons have to do with tears?

James Kavanaugh

Should I Use the Same Baby Clothes?

Remember all those baby clothes you accumulated in anticipation of your new baby's arrival? You probably stored them away after your baby died until the next time. Well, the next time is here and now you need to decide what to do with all those cute outfits. When you bring them out of storage and check each one over to make sure it is just right for this baby, the memories will come flooding in stronger than you may expect. You'll remember how cute your baby looked or would have looked. You'll remember the baby shower that was attended by your friends who were also excited about your becoming a mother. You'll remember how positive everyone was that everything would be all right. Don't be surprised if the tears come pouring forth. Some women find they can get only one drawer of clothes ready at a time, before the pain becomes too acute. And some have asked a close friend to help in order to lighten the pain a bit.

The decision whether or not to use these clothes for your new baby may or may not be a problem for you. On the one hand, putting the clothes on your new baby may seem the natural thing to do. After all, you would have passed these clothes on to your next child if this child hadn't died. The idea seems reasonable and practical. It relieves the family of the financial burden of buying a whole new wardrobe.

On the other hand you may want to put away the "very special" outfits as keepsakes and use only the other clothes. Or if it is just too painful to think of putting your dead child's clothes on another child — if you find yourself focusing on the clothes and what your dead child, rather than your new child, would have looked like in them, you need to give yourself permission to put the clothes away. Why not exchange them with another mother who had a baby die, or a pregnant friend? That way you can have "new" clothes without having to spend money. Or a resale shop may be willing to swap outfits with you.

Some mothers say that they enjoy seeing the clothes on their new baby and that they know that their dead baby would approve.

Preparing for Labor and Birth

If you took prepared childbirth classes during your last pregnancy you may have found them very helpful. On the other hand you may have felt that they gave an unrealistic picture of what you were about to experience. Two commonly heard complaints from bereaved parents are that their childbirth classes did not give enough attention to pain in childbirth and to the possibility of the death of the baby.

If you thought the classes were going to teach you how to avoid pain altogether during labor and birth you were probably very disillusioned. Most women after going through labor, no matter how well prepared they were, acknowledge that there was pain in childbirth. Indeed a measure of pain and a lot of hard work are to be regarded as a necessary part of the birth experience. However, how one views the pain makes a big difference in whether the experience is remembered as positive or negative. This is not to suggest that you should somehow treasure the discomfort of your birth experience or relish the role of martyr, but only that you can come to appreciate pain because of lessons it may teach you. This is an issue for many childbearing couples, not just bereaved parents.

But it is difficult, if not impossible, to imagine how a woman could have appreciation for the pain of childbirth after she has suffered the death of her child at or before birth. What's the value of all that pain when there is nothing to show for it? Instead, bereaved parents have told us, "The birth experience is not what people make it out to be. I am no longer looking forward to any wonderful, shared birth experience. All I want is a live baby."

Parents also report feelings of resentment that at no time during their childbirth classes was death ever talked about as even a remote possibility. Given such feelings it is no wonder that bereaved parents have difficulty sitting in a class with 10 "untouched," naive couples who are anticipating a childbirth filled with bliss. Though educators are beginning to agree that death and grief are valid topics for discussion in classes it is difficult for some of them to discuss these topics for fear of upsetting the parents.

Our experience with bereaved parents has shown otherwise. In fact most bereaved parents are relieved to be able to discuss their secret fears, to know that they will not be abandoned if something tragic happens and to have some sense of how to handle the situation if it happens to them or to someone they know.

If you are a bereaved parent, we know that your previous experience will cloud your present one, and that your aspirations for this subsequent birth experience may have you in turmoil. You may have no desire to have to deal with pain, but on the other hand you may be anxious about taking pain medications because of the possible harmful effects to your baby. Then again, you may still want to achieve natural birth with no medications. You may find yourself intellectualizing one approach but doing the exact opposite. For example, one woman we know whose stillbirth was by cesarean section, wanted a vaginal birth for her subsequent pregnancy. She did fine holding on to that plan until the 39th week when she couldn't contain her anxieties any longer. She requested a cesarean birth. Another woman wanted no drugs during labor but found herself so nervous and unable to relax that she needed large amounts of analgesia to make it through the birth.

But in spite of your difficult history, there are things that you can do to make your subsequent birth as special as possible. You do not need to look upon labor as a necessary evil nor do you need to let your labor be governed by an embittered past. And you are capable of facing the natural discomforts of pregnancy without a lot of interventions if you choose to.

Now what does all that mean? It means simply that you will not be able to adopt a story book approach to this birth. But it doesn't mean that you shouldn't attempt to achieve the kind of birth experience that you value for yourself. If having a vaginal, unmedicated birth remains important to you, it is still very possible. You just need to plan for it differently than before. If you aren't overly concerned about the effects of medication and their normal use during labor and delivery then you will do okay too. If you had a cesarean birth before, and want a vaginal birth with this baby, that may very well be an obtainable goal. But we also think that, if you had a previous cesarean birth, it is reasonable for you to want to choose that type of birth experience this time. The key here is not to set yourself up to fail at something that is important to you. That way you won't have to deal with grief over lost expectations after this baby is born. Now that you know some of the potential roadblocks you can prepare for them.

Suggestions

1. If you can't bring yourself to go to regular classes, find a childbirth educator who is willing to tutor you. The ideal situation would be a group of people with similar experiences where you all "know" the broad range of possible outcomes. Here you can be open about your fears but at the same time help each other to be hopeful.
2. Concentrate on learning how to relax. Relaxation, understanding how your body works and allowing the process to take its course are fundamental to being able to deal with the rigors of childbirth.
3. Adopt the idea that the labor contractions are the work that your body has to go through in order to deliver your baby. The harder the work that is being done, the closer you are to being finished.

"The sound of my baby's heart beat on the fetal monitor was music to my ears. I know the persistent sound was annoying everyone else though."

"Every time I would turn, or the baby would move, and the monitor didn't register the baby's heart beat, I would panic. I needed to hear the sound of my baby all the time."

"The nurse would come in and reassure me that everything was all right. After she left I would turn to my husband and ask him if he thought she was telling the truth."

"Just as they were about to begin the cesarean section I thought about the extramarital affair I had had several years ago and wondered if I would be punished again for that mistake. I don't really believe that God punishes people in that way, but I still thought about it."

"I didn't want to push. I didn't want the pregnancy to end. As long as I was still pregnant I didn't have to face the truth that there might be something wrong with this baby too."

"I was desperate to get this baby born, but scared to death to have it born. I wondered, 'Am I really cut out to be a mother?'"

"The birth of our son was a draining experience for all of us. The doctors kept trying to give my wife medication. She withdrew from everybody, into her own private world. The nurses were exhausted from trying to make things okay for us. After it was over one of the nurses commented on how difficult a birth it had been and asked how I felt about it. I looked at her in amazement. 'Difficult?' I asked. 'This was nothing. You should have been here the last time. **At least this time we got a live baby.'** I guess it all depends on your perspective."

"My oldest son had died only a few hours before I went into labor with this baby. I couldn't care less about the outcome. I didn't care if I lived or died."

"The nurses kept urging me to look into the mirror so I could see my baby be born. I didn't want to look in case she was dead. Later when I saw the pictures I was glad that I hadn't looked. She was blue in the pictures. I wasn't prepared for that."

"He didn't cry immediately. The only sound I could hear was my own heart beat."

The Challenge of Labor

The time has come at last — the end of a long journey toward parenthood. For some of you this will be the climax of many months filled with memories of pregnancy and grief. Finally you will have something to show for your courageous efforts.

If you are like most pregnant women, bereaved or not, you will be wishing that the baby could arrive two weeks early rather than two weeks late. Even if you worked hard at not succumbing to unnecessary medical intervention during this pregnancy (in order to reassure yourself that everything was all right with your baby), you may find yourself greatly tempted at this point to get the jump on nature and opt for induced labor. This pregnancy has gone on long enough. You know that the baby — at 37 to 43 weeks — is now within the normal time frame for an uncomplicated birth. You may feel you've waited long enough for the opportunity to hold this baby in your arms, and that you have exhausted all your resources for keeping your sanity in check.

Your anxieties about the birth will probably be heightened at this point. Because you live your life through your past experiences you will recall each stage of your previous labor as you go through the process over again. Your situation is very similar to that of a person who has been in a traffic accident. The first time you pass the intersection where the accident occurred you will remember everything. You may even break out in a cold sweat. Each time you travel that same road, your memory of the experience will fade a little more until one day you will pass the spot without even thinking of the accident until you are far down the road. In the same way your anxieties about this birth will tend to diminish as you face them squarely. The more times you can review the previous labor, by talking it through, or visiting the hospital where it took place, the less emotional turmoil you will have to experience when you are in labor this time. No, you won't forget completely, but the memory will not be as likely to overwhelm you, if you prepare for it.

Plan to make several trips to the hospital before your due date. The first time you may just want to drive to the area and then take a leisurely walk around the hospital grounds. The next time go inside and register for your hospital stay. Plan to make one of your trips at a time when you can see the babies in the nursery. Next it will be time to return to the labor and delivery area. Many hospitals offer tours to pregnant families. Even if you've taken the tour in the past do it again. And finally, you may want to make an appointment with the head nurse in labor and delivery.

Ask yourself these questions before your meeting with the head nurse:

1. Do you want to be placed in a labor and delivery room different from the one where you were before?
2. Do you want to be cared for by the same nurse that was with you the last time?
3. Do you want to hold the baby immediately after birth?
4. Do you want to observe the birth?
5. Do you want to have a pediatrician in attendance at the birth?
6. Do you want rooming-in or do you want your baby cared for in the nursery and brought to you only occasionally?

Talk to the nurse about what you think will be most helpful to you to make this birth as easy as possible.

Sometimes it is helpful to write out specific requests and mail these to the hospital, in care of the maternity section. That way the information will be on hand when you arrive, in case your birth happens at a time when the head nurse is not around. A word of caution though: the written word can be misinterpreted. Be as clear and specific as you can. And be careful to choose wording that will not offend the nursing staff and make it harder for them to care for you.

Courage is doing what you are afraid to do.

Edie Rickenbacker

You've been through labor before, so you know it's not a picnic, but depending upon the outcome and the extent of the medical interventions during your previous labor and delivery you may have a distorted picture of what your birth experience will be like under "normal" conditions.

For example, if your previous pregnancy resulted in a miscarriage or premature birth you may not fully expect the physical discomfort that you are likely to encounter in a full term birth. We wish we could assure you that your next birth will be at least as easy as the earlier one, but to do so would be unfair to you. The contractions you experienced last time only needed to be strong enough to open the cervix a few centimeters, because your baby weighed only a few ounces or pounds. But in order to deliver a full term baby (usually between six and eight pounds) the contractions must be strong enough to dilate the cervix to ten centimeters.

On the other hand, if your last birth was at full term and

physically painful, complicated by the strain of knowing that your baby was already dead, or in grave danger, you may have greatly exaggerated fears about what lies ahead for you. Emotional pain increases physical pain. In fact this next labor and delivery may turn out to be easier than you have imagined, if you have done a thorough job of dealing with the emotional pain ahead of time.

Labor and grief are very similar. Both can be considered primary functions. A primary function is an activity that demands your undivided attention. In other words, you can handle only one primary function at a time with efficiency. Doing anything else while you are engaged in a primary function will be very distracting, and most likely irritating, to you. You can wash the dishes while holding a conversation with someone, and most of the time you can drive a car while listening to the radio because normally these are not primary functions. But if while driving and listening you suddenly find yourself in a heavy downpour of rain so that you can hardly see the center strip on the road, you may have to turn off the radio so you can concentrate better. Your driving has become a primary function. You don't want to be distracted by the radio while trying to steer the car. For some people, watching television is a primary function. They get so absorbed by what they're watching that it is impossible to converse with them about anything until they turn off the set. Conversation with them is impossible.

When you are in active labor little things can be very distracting to you. This is also true during the grief process. Remember how hard it was to concentrate on other things when you were preoccupied with your loss in the early days in your grief?

Grief has been described as labor-in-reverse. The first part of labor is generally mild and manageable. At this stage it is nice, but not necessary, to have others around. You won't lose control if they happen to step out of the room for a while. But as labor progresses it becomes harder to stay in control. You need other people's love and support to keep going.

The picture of grief is just the opposite. At first you feel like you are holding on for dear life, and you need to be reminded constantly that you're not going crazy. Thoughts of your dead child fill your entire day. But as the weeks and months pass by, the sharp emotional pains get more bearable and you don't need the constant support from those around you. The world starts to come back into focus again.

If you haven't dealt with your grief, you may find that labor will trigger grief again. And during your labor you will find yourself confronted with both grieving and laboring at the same time. All those memories of the last time that you had so carefully tucked away so you wouldn't have to feel pain are now likely to surface.

The past is filled with lessons for the future. Don't be afraid to learn them.

Suggestions for labor

Try to make your baby's birth as special as possible. Even though at this point in your life just making it through may be enough, try to think of things that will make this birth something very positive to be able to look back on. Some day your child will want to know how you celebrated his birth.

1. Consider having a special friend or relative with you and your partner during labor. One that you've shared your joys and fears of this pregnancy with and who can be supportive of both of your emotional needs. Check with your doctor or hospital to see if there are any special arrangements you have to make in order to have an additional person with you. It is possible that you will have a number of people who will want to be at your baby's birth. Some of them have been waiting a long time for this baby too. But it's important that you protect yourself from having to take care of everyone else's needs right now and just tend to yourselves. Many women have commented that though it was wonderful to have the love and support around them they felt they were having to perform for others.

2. Consider taking pictures of the birth so you will have some tangible evidence of the event. Women who have had pictures taken have found the pictures to be extremely helpful as they tried to recapture parts of their birth, but couldn't remember because they were either too afraid to look or were too busy birthing. In case you are one who decides not to look, you may grateful to be able to "see" after it's all over. Even the most modest of women have treasured these pictures.

3. You may want to record on tape the last few minutes of the birth so you can capture your baby's first cries and your first comments.

4. Plan a birthday party for this little baby's entrance. No need to wait for a first birthday, have it now.

Considering how dangerous everything is nothing is really very frightening
Gertrude Stein

Holly's Ashes

I remember very well the day we buried Holly's ashes on Neakahni Mountain. Mike had discovered the place and shown it to me years earlier. We stood on the cliff's edge and watched the waves crashing on the jagged rocks hundreds of feet below. The horizon was before us and a cascading waterfall behind us. It was as if we were standing on the edge of the world with nature's majesty surrounding us. To us it seemed the most beautiful spot on earth. That was the way we remembered it . . . always during the warmth of summer.

As we discussed what should be done with our daughter's ashes, the memory of this place came to me. Of course, it seemed the only place for a baby to be. We bought a tiny teddy bear to keep her company on her journey. It also seemed important to leave flowers on the grave, pink of course. So we started our trek to the cliff's edge with hiking boots, shovel, flowers and bear and that tiny gold foil box marked "cremated remains of Holly Beth Stanbro." I remember staring at those words, at that box, with anger in my heart. I had just given birth to a baby and this is all that I have to show for it.

It was quite a different place in the cold months of winter. Very few people visited the spot at that time of year and the growth was dense and difficult to make our way through. There was a cold drizzle falling and a bitter wind, cold and relentless. The grass was brown, the trees bare of foliage. The ocean seemed gray and stormy. The place seemed barren, desolate. How fitting. I felt desolate, cold and barren. The whole world seemed dead — and so was our daughter.

When we finished the deed we stood embracing, weeping and strong in each other's arms. This was so crazy, our world was all mixed up. We had just given birth yet here we stood beside a grave.

We couldn't have known then that the following spring Matthew would be born. What a joyous time it would be for us. What a miracle that this baby would be born alive and healthy. His cries were lusty, his movements strong, his body perfect. I can still hear my doctor calling out, "He has hair!" This doctor had seen me through the tragedy of Holly's death and was now genuinely elated at the birth of a healthy son. Mike had given me a gardenia in a dish in my room.

When my doctor visited me one morning he was overwhelmed by the fragrance and said, "Oh that smell . . . I thought I was in heaven." I replied, "You are."

We visited Holly's grave for the first time on the Memorial Day following Matthew's birth. It was one of the first warm days of spring. Matthew was about six weeks old, and while we still missed Holly, we were delighted with our new little son. So off we went again, hiking boots, flowers and Matthew in a Snugli. Erik brought up the rear as four-year-olds do.

I couldn't help noticing the striking contrast to our last visit to the spot, the day we had buried Holly. The sun was shining and a warm breeze blew. The grass was green and the wildflowers were in bloom. So many colors — purple, yellow, white and red — and the spot seemed vibrant and beautiful once again. Next to my heart slept Matthew, completely oblivious to the joy he had brought to us. I could feel Holly's presence. Did she know we had come? Did she know we had brought her brothers? As I looked around at the beauty of the spot, I realized that we had come full circle. The world was alive again.

Barbara Stanbro

Chapter 5
Beyond Birth

Terrible Two

I thought it was over,
The crushing pain.
The memories were sweeter.
Only a little twinge now and then . . .
Only a few tears
When I thought too much
Of what I was missing . . .
My little girl.
I didn't expect these birthday blues,
These tears, this hurt, the regrets.
It's terrible.
She would have been two.

Barbara Stanbro

"I couldn't imagine letting the nurses give my baby sugar water so I could sleep. There is going to be a time when I won't be able to hold him. I want to make use of the time I have now. I live regretting that I did not use all the time that I could have with my baby that died."

Husband to wife: "You cried when you came home after your baby died, and now you come home with a live baby and still you cry. Isn't there anything that will make you happy?"

"I was absolutely elated. She was beautiful. But about two hours later when I was settled in my postpartum room and everyone had gone home I cried for my baby that had died."

"I didn't think of anything. I wasn't happy. I wasn't sad. I was just relieved the pregnancy was over."

"The doctor said she was alive and I kept saying, no, I know she's dead. I'd fall asleep and wake up a few minutes later and again ask what I had and if she was dead. I'm sure my husband and doctor must have been terribly frustrated with me."

"We were absolutely overwhelmed with fear that this baby was going to die too when he had to be admitted to the NICU because of jaundice. The nurses couldn't understand why we were acting this way. They kept telling us that jaundice was no big deal and that all the other babies in the unit were much sicker than ours. Our first baby wasn't supposed to die either."

"We decorated the nursery real cute, but she has yet to sleep in it. She is always in the same room that I am in At night she sleeps with us. I am too afraid to have her sleep that far away from me."

"We were both exhausted from having the baby in bed with us all night. My husband said she had to sleep in her own room. I reluctantly gave in and put her in her own room. I was exhausted the next day from lying awake all night listening to make sure she was all right."

"I think we just have to accept that we will be preoccupied with our baby's health for awhile. If he cries we're distracted and if he seems too quiet we're worried."

"Even after our son was born I continued to cling to and grieve for our daughter until we found out our son needed surgery. All of a sudden it struck me that my daughter was just fine wherever she is. My living son was the one that needed me to be concerned about him, not my dead daughter."

"Before my grief was from longing for what I thought would be. Now my grief is real, because now I know what I lost."

Evelyn's Story

My daughter, Emily, was born with critical aortic stenosis, a congenital heart defect. When she was 14 days old, she underwent an emergency valvectomy. Jeff and I were told that she would need two more surgeries to get her grown up into young adulthood.

I spent the first year of Emily's life grieving over the loss of a healthy child. I could not believe that this terrible thing had happened to me — to my daughter.

I loved Emily as I had never loved anyone before. Each day, each moment with her seemed so precious. I knew her life was not to be taken for granted. When Emily was nearly two years old the need for further surgery became apparent. The correct size homograph needed to be located. After a few months of waiting, Emily underwent surgery to replace her defective valve. The trauma to her heart was too much for the delicate organ to bear. She died on November 15, 1987.

I suffered through two excruciating months — days filled with gut-wrenching, heart-breaking pain, long periods when I felt that life was not worth living, when it took all my strength just to rise from my bed to face another day without Emily. When all I could see ahead of me was the darkest of darkness, I discovered that I was pregnant again.

I felt shocked, invaded, unprepared, overwhelmed and really out of control. I was beset with morning sickness. Already consumed by my grief so that I felt I had nothing more to give, a new life had suddenly appeared to demand more of me.

Having already had the experience of caring for an infant, I knew that there would be limited time for myself, after the baby came. I believed also that we would be faced with new and unanticipated grief issues with the birth of this next baby. And so I felt an urgency about my grief.

My life became a balancing act. I had to figure out how to eat properly, rest to relieve the fatigue, take walks to care for both my mind and my body, make time to express my ever-present burden of sorrow, and try to come up with some "good stuff" mentally for the baby.

I often felt guilty that I had so few positive feelings to offer to this new little one. In contrast to the pregnancy with Emily I had to work hard at wanting this new child. The pain of losing Emily was too intense — too real — to want to risk my heart again so soon.

Nearly all of our family and friends were openly excited and happy about my pregnancy. But excitement and joy had disappeared from my life the day Emily died, and the excitement and joy did not suddenly reappear simply because I was pregnant. It was Emily I wanted, with all my heart and soul, not this other baby. It all felt like too much too soon. I hated other people for being happy and I resented the suggestion that I ought to be happy too.

Because the baby's due date was just three weeks after what would have been Emily's third birthday, I spent the entire pregnancy hoping that the baby would not be born early. But Emily's birthday came and went with all the trappings customary for such occasions. The final evening of the month came and I breathed a sign of relief. I felt lucky knowing that at least this baby could have a different birth month from that of Emily. That next morning I was awakened by a labor pain.

Though pre-natal testing indicated I was carrying a healthy baby it was difficult to believe that another tragedy was not awaiting us. I also found it difficult not to resent the easy reassurances offered by friends and family, who told me that everything was going to turn out all right.

All during the delivery, my mind was filled with Emily. My feelings for my daughter made it hard for me to focus on the work I needed to do to bring this new baby into the world. I could think only of how I missed Emily, and how much I wanted her rather than this baby I didn't know, and whom I was afraid to love.

Later, at home, we were surprised at how the presence of this new baby amplified our sense of Emily's absence. The house seemed so lonely, so empty without the little family member who should have been there — running around with excitement at having a brother. The perception of the incompleteness of our family fell heavy on our hearts.

Again our friends, neighbors and family expressed happiness at the news of this new birth. And again, in contrast to their feelings, I experienced sadness, guilt, and inadequacy. Although I was truly grateful for a healthy son and an "uncomplicated" pregnancy and birth, I longed for my fair-haired Emily. I was not able to be happy and sad at the same time. I was sad because I realized that Ryan would not know his sister, EVER. Ryan could not fill the void in my life left by Emily's death.

And I felt alone. It seemed that, except for Jeff, I was the only one still missing Emily. Rarely did anyone mention her name to me.

Now that Ryan has been with me for several months, I've noticed that it occurs to me often that this little person could also die. I sometimes run into his room anticipating the worst. For this reason it has been harder to fall in love with Ryan than it was with Emily. However, we survived the death of our daughter, so I knew we could survive this new challenge. By taking one day at a time, by juggling needs, and by communicating with each other, Jeff and I have lived through another difficult period in our lives.

Our grief, and the methods we use to move with it and through it, are indeed quite different. It's taken hours of effort on both of our parts to keep our relationship a functioning one. We've learned things about each other and about ourselves we wish we had never had to know. Our lives have changed dramatically since the death of our daughter Emily. We've learned that we are powerless when it comes to certain life events. We've learned that it really makes no difference how hard we've tried, or how good we are or have been, we can't bring Emily back. WE CAN'T REPLACE HER. We can only make choices about our future.

And you know, that little Ryan is worming his way into my heart.

Evelyn Taylor

Postpartum Days

Most subsequent parents imagine, or at least hope, that their lives will be happy again once the new baby is born. Friends, relatives, and caregivers also assume this. Unfortunately, this longed for happiness is rarely automatic or immediate. You may find the early days postpartum similar to a roller coaster ride with lots of highs and lows as you work through ambivalent and sometimes confusing feelings about your new role. You face a complex puzzle: how does one maintain the role of the bereaved parent while also being a new parent at the same time? How convenient it would be if you could just shed the old role of bereaved parent like a winter coat now that spring has come. But it's unrealistic and certainly unfair to expect that a little baby will be able to take away all the pain of your previous loss. Only you can resolve that.

Sometimes parents will also find they are still waiting for something catastrophic to happen to the new baby, and so the anxiety of being hurt again remains. Passing the point in the pregnancy where disaster struck the last time will bring little comfort to you. You may then find yourself preoccupied with concerns about your baby's exposure to childhood diseases, or about the possibility of sudden infant death syndrome. Or you may worry that your baby has some congenital problem that has yet to be diagnosed.

During the early days following your return from the hospital you may find yourself continually on the verge of tears — tears of joy and tears of sadness. The intensity of your emotions comes from many sources. Some of it may be caused from the release of tension that has been building up over the past nine months, or from the hormonal changes that are happening in your body. Insufficient sleep, a common problem to new parents, most likely plays a factor in your emotions too, as does the added burden of coming to terms with how your relationship with this baby affects your relationship with the one that died.

Three things are essential to help you make it through these days. The first is a pediatrician or family physician whom you know to be competent, and whom you feel comfortable calling. You will probably need lots of reassurances that those "little things" that you are concerned about will not be taken lightly.

Second, you need a friend in whom you can confide. Another bereaved parent, or a close friend who has seen you through the difficult days of grief may fit this role. There may be days when you won't like this new baby because he doesn't measure up to your expectations of a perfect baby. Remember, only dead babies are perfect babies. They're only perfect because they never got the chance to keep you up at night or have colic. But it will be good for you to talk about it. You might find it hard to admit this to your mother if you assume she would think you were being ungrateful. This is also humbling if you have only recently been saying, while in the throes of grief, "At least your baby is alive. I'd give anything if my baby just had colic. I'd walk the floor for a month and love every moment of it." Even one understanding, non-judgmental friend can do wonders for your sanity. Most mothers have these negative feelings at times.

The third essential is to be kind to yourself. Give yourself permission to be a little crazy for a while. Let others pamper you. In time, as you finish letting go of your baby that died, you will begin to be more comfortable with the new role of parenting this baby.

Yes, you will feel the joy that comes with all new life, but it will be different from the joy of your untouched sisters. Where theirs is naive and light, yours will be seasoned with truth and wisdom.

Two Flowers

Two flowers in our vase
The first of delicate silk
forever a bud about to open
The second of nature's fabric
a bud about to open and hopefully
unfold into a blossom full fragranced
of multiple hue and layers
that in time will fade
and gracefully drop its petals.

Deborah Carpenter

Dear Linnea,

Three years since you appeared, and
disappeared so quickly . . .
You'd be filling the forest with
your shouts of laughter and wonder;
You'd be begging to go down to the
river and dip your feet in its
icy waters;
You'd be tickling and tugging
and teaching all kinds of things
to your baby sister, Jenna . . .

The sister who will never know you,
and yet, through us, will know of
your love, your spirit, which is
with us still
   (and always will be).

The tears don't come as often these
days (but the times they do, when I'm
alone, they wrench through my soul
like a twisting knife. I wonder
whether they'll ever stop. They do
   for now).

The pain of your unexpected leave-
taking isn't so intense these days,
but it pops up, equally as unexpected . . .
When the sun beams down on your sister's
hair, and I see you (and remember . . .)
When your sister snuggles up to your
dad, and I see him holding you close
that first time (and remember . . .)
When I pull something out of the drawer
that was given for you (and remember . . .)
When the month of your birth and death
approaches and my bittersweet memories
awaken, I see you (and remember . . .)

Our pain has brought us closer to the
universal pain that everyone suffers . . .
It has taught us to be a little more
accepting, a bit more empathetic.

It is still teaching us as we
remember you with love, dear Linnea.
                    Barbara Steltz-Fahlander

115

Bibliography:

To our knowledge there are no other books in print that deal specifically with subsequent pregnancies. However there are many books that may be helpful to you in your situation either by providing medical information or by helping you to interpret what you are feeling. Reading can be a powerful ally, answering some of your technical questions and helping you to discover how normal and natural are your responses and reactions in the context of pregnancy and grief.

1. *Parental Infant Bonding,* by Marshall Klaus and John Kennel, is an in-depth study of parental behavior and how family ties begin. The first edition of this book was the first to acknowledge the grief of parents following a stillbirth.

2. *Transitions,* by William Bridges, deals with strategies for coping with difficult, painful and confusing life situations. Every personal change brings with it new fears and further confusion. This book helps us to learn how to handle 'endings' and 'beginnings' in our lives.

3. *Making Love During Pregnancy,* by Elizabeth Bing and Libby Coleman, is a refreshing and open reference to sex during the childbearing year. This illustrated book helps dispel myths that may encumber your sexuality during pregnancy.

4. *New Hope for Problem Pregnancies,* by Robert Creasy and Diane Hales, gives information on screening and monitoring techniques, new drugs and new technologies which help to recognize risks, detect problems and treat sick babies before birth.

5. *The Safe Pregnancy Book,* by Carol Ann Rinzler, is a well-researched and comprehensive book covering information necessary to make informed choices about your habits and environment that may affect your unborn child.

6. *The Dream Worlds of Pregnancy,* by Eileen Stukane, is a helpful guide to couples interested in putting their "night time work" to good use during the day. For those who aren't afraid to try to understand what happens to us in the realm of the unconscious the book will be very helpful.

7. *After a Loss in Pregnancy,* by Nancy Berezin, is an excellent source for the bereaved parent, offering both comfort in the wake of grief and technical information to help you better understand the medical reasons for a pregnancy loss.

8. *The Penguin Adoption Handbook,* by Edmund Blair Bolles, offers step-by-step suggestions for working with adoption agencies. The author respects the need for counseling, support and advice throughout the adoption process.

9. *The Complete Book of Pregnancy and Childbirth,* by Sheila Kitzinger, covers a wide range of important information for you including fetal growth and development, general emotional changes associated with pregnancy, and down-to-earth suggestions for coping with labor and birth.

10. *Getting Pregnant and Staying Pregnant,* a guide to infertility and high risk pregnancy, by Diana Raab, is a good resource, easily understandable and sensitive in its portrayal of "hard times and decisions."

The following is a list of mail order book stores that carry a large variety of bereavement literature.

Birth and Life Bookstore
7001 Alonzo Ave. N.W.
P.O. Box 70625
Seattle, WA 98107-0625

Centering Corporation
P.O. Box 3367
Omaha, NE 68103

ICEA Bookcenter
P.O. Box 20048
Minneapolis, MN 55420

National organizations that may be able to put you in touch with a parent support group in your area are:

Compassionate Friends
National Office
P.O. Box 3696
Oak Brook, IL 60522-3696

S.H.A.R.E.
St. Elizabeth Hospital
211 S. Third Street
Bellville, IL 62222

U.N.I.T.E.
c/o Jeanes Hospital
7600 Central Ave.
Philadelphia, PA 19111

In order to have
    a successful relationship
you need to put out of your mind
any lessons learned
    from previous relationships
because if you carry
    a sensitivity or fear with you
you won't be acting freely
and you won't let yourself
    be really known

In order to have
    a successful relationship
it is essential that both people
be completely open and honest
                    Susan Polis Schutz

Epilogue

Buried within the pain of your child's death lies a gift for you. You may not be ready to accept that now, but you must trust that some good will come out of your child's short journey. Sometimes it's hard to see the gift if you feel you must hold tight to your grief, or are inclined to deny that anything significant happened to you as a result of your baby's death. You have learned much about death. These lessons will teach you about life. You alone will choose whether or not you will face life boldly and joyfully after defeat. We wish you the courage and peace to choose life.

Will we forget . . . no never
But we don't need to.
We've loved
We've cared
We've cried
We've grown
And now it's time to smile again.

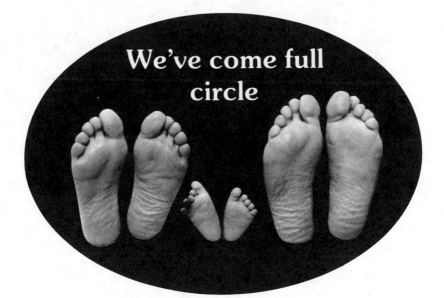

We've come full circle